Manual of Gastroenterologic Procedures

Third Edition

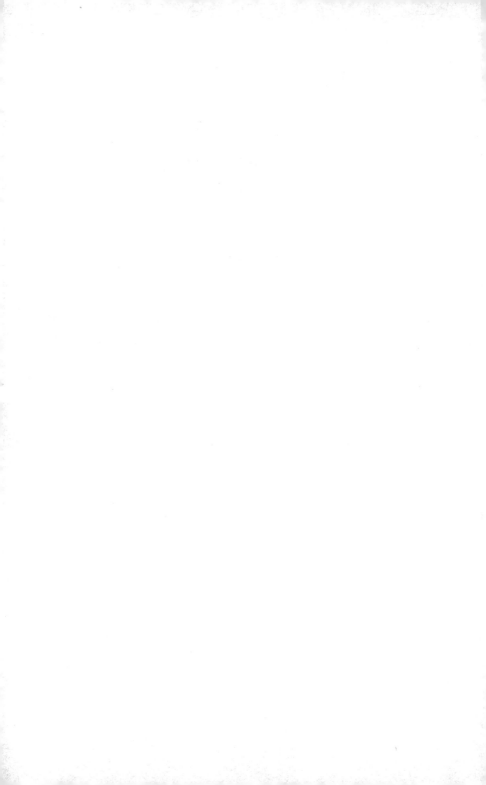

Manual of Gastroenterologic Procedures

Third Edition

Editor

Douglas A. Drossman, M.D.

Professor
Division of Digestive Diseases
University of North Carolina School of Medicine
Chapel Hill, North Carolina

Raven Press New York

Raven Press, Ltd., 1185 Avenue of the Americas, New York, New York 10036

Made in the United States of America

Library of Congress Cataloging-in-Publication Data

Manual of gastroenterologic procedures / editor, Douglas A. Drossman.
— 3rd ed.
    p.   cm.
  Includes bibliographical references and index.
  ISBN 0-88167-944-5
    1. Gastroenterology—Methodology—Handbooks, manuals, etc.
  I. Drossman, Douglas A.
    [DNLM: 1. Gastroenterology—handbooks. WI 39 M294]
  RC802.M35   1992
  616.3'3—dc20
  DNLM/DLC
  for Library of Congress   92-17142
                                                                  CIP

9   8   7   6   5   4   3

In honor of the retirement of John T. Sessions, Jr., M.D., the distinguished founder of our Division. Dr. Sessions remains a continual source of guidance, support, and inspiration for all of us.

In memory of Oscar L. Sapp III, M.D., a devoted and respected member of our division for eighteen years.

Contents

Needles

Diagnostic Endoscopy

Procedures for Pediatric Patients

Contributors

Eugene M. Bozymski, M.D.
Donald P. Brannan, M.D.
Douglas A. Drossman, M.D.
William D. Heizer, M.D.
Kim L. Isaacs, M.D., Ph.D.
Ray L. James, Jr., M.D.
Kenneth B. Klein, M.D.
Henry R. Lesesne, M.D.
Sidney L. Levinson, M.D.

C. Thomas Nuzum, M.D.
Roy C. Orlando, M.D.
Don W. Powell, M.D.
Meredith P. Reinhold,
  R.N., C.G.C.
Robert S. Sandler, M.D., Ph.D.
R. Balfour Sartor, M.D.
Martin H. Ulshen, M.D.
John I. Wurzelmann, M.D.

The contributors are, or have been, members of the Division of Digestive Diseases, University of North Carolina School of Medicine, Chapel Hill, North Carolina. Dr. Ulshen is Chief of the Division of Pediatric Gastroenterology at the University of North Carolina; Drs. Levinson and James, respectively, are in private practice in Chapel Hill, North Carolina, and Newport News, Virginia; Dr. Orlando is Chief of Gastroenterology at Tulane University Medical School; and Dr. Powell is Chairman of the Department of Medicine, The University of Texas at Galveston.

xi

Preface

It is with great pleasure that we offer this third edition of *Manual of Gastroenterologic Procedures* from the Division of Digestive Diseases at the University of North Carolina School of Medicine. As with the previous editions, our goal is to provide a resource for physicians, nurses, technicians, and students in most of the gastroenterological procedures. The information is presented in a standardized, yet straightforward format that highlights the indications, contraindications, patient preparation, techniques, and complications for 40 procedures. In addition to a section on the organization and function of the procedure unit itself, the chapters are conveniently organized into sections on tubes, needles, diagnostic endoscopy, therapeutic endoscopy, and pediatric procedures.

The manual can serve as a supplement to more comprehensive endoscopy manuals. Here, the endoscopic sections provide a "quick look," with essential information and helpful tips (for example, what to do when the sphincterotome will not advance into the common duct). In addition, about half of the chapters are devoted to important nonendoscopic procedures (e.g., insertion of Minnesota tube, esophageal and rectal manometry, liver biopsy, paracentesis, and feeding tube intubation) that are not easily found in one book.

Several changes have been made to reflect the advances in gastroenterological practice over the past five years. New chapters include ambulatory intraesophageal pH monitoring, laser therapy, and a section devoted to medications used in the procedure unit (conscious sedation, topical anesthetics, motility/anti-motility drugs, antibiotics for bacterial endocarditis prophylaxis, and biliary tract manipulation). Several chapters have been extensively revised. We have updated the section on naso/gastrointestinal intubation to include newer devices, and describe the endoscopic rather than capsule technique for small bowel biopsy (the capsule technique is included in the pediatric section). We have also added injection therapy to the chapter on ablation of bleeding gastrointestinal lesions, describe both the one-step and three-step method for balloon dilatation of strictures, and we have included a discussion on the use of dual (radiologic/endoscopic) biliary stent placement.

We trust that this third edition will continue to serve many purposes for all of us involved in the diagnosis and care of patients with gastrointestinal disorders.

Douglas A. Drossman, M.D.

Acknowledgment

The authors would like to thank Peter G. Bedick for his assistance in providing the illustrations.

The Procedure Unit

Meredith P. Reinhold

Based on our experience at a tertiary-care medical center, this chapter offers guidelines for the establishment, organization, and management of a gastrointestinal (GI) procedure unit. Our recommendations can be adapted for use in private practice settings. The primary focus should be to create an environment in which patient needs can be met in a safe, efficient, cost-effective, and concerned manner.

Location and Characteristics of the Unit

The procedure unit should be located in an area of the hospital readily accessible to outpatients. The size of the unit, its equipment, and furnishings will depend on patient volume and the types of procedures anticipated. Physical separation of the clinical area from the administrative and waiting areas is advisable; attention should be paid to sound reduction and to the flow of traffic.

Procedure Room Equipment and Supplies in Procedure Rooms

1. The room should be organized with the bed as its activity center (1). A comfortable and well-designed procedure bed with bed rails and raising, lowering, tilting, and wheel-locking capabilities is recommended. When needed, the bed should be able to accommodate C-arm fluoroscopy.
2. The spatial arrangement of the room should allow for turning the bed within the room, for wheelchair or transport stretcher entry, and for crash cart use.
3. Intravenous (i.v.) ceiling tracks and hangers. Curtain tracks

1

should be within the room to provide patient privacy when the door is opened.

4. Video endoscopy cart with processor, light source if needed, and photographic, data entry, and electrocautery equipment.
5. Video monitors properly placed for ease of viewing (2).
6. Patient monitors for blood pressure, pulse, and oxygen saturation. An available cardiac monitor with printout capability is also recommended.
7. Counter space should be available opposite the physician and video cart.
8. Wall suction, oxygen outlets, and oxygen administration equipment.
9. There should be adequate ventilation, with a room thermostat.
10. Rheostat-controlled lighting.
11. X-ray view boxes.
12. Shelving with gowns, gloves, masks, and goggles near room entry.
13. Hand-washing sink.
14. Available emergency drugs should include naloxone hydrochloride (Narcan), atropine, diphenhydramine hydrochloride (Benadryl), epinephrine, and fluazemil, along with the usual i.v. supplies.
15. In-room supplies include: patient preparation materials, linen supply and hamper, foot stool, rolling stool, trash receptacle, adequate cabinetry, biological specimen collection supplies, needle disposal containers, telephone, intercom system, and clock.

Equipment and Supplies Adjacent to Procedure Rooms

1. Adjoining or adjacent patient toilet facilities.
2. Clinical hopper for disposal of biological wastes.
3. Wheelchair-capacity dressing room with toilet facilities, lockers, hand-washing sink, linen shelving and hamper, sitting bench, call bell, and handrails.
4. Cardiopulmonary resuscitation cart and defibrillator.

5. Storage area for traveling endoscopy cart.
6. Storage closets/areas for unit supplies, linen cart, endoscope cases, and mailing cartons. (Store one original mailing carton for each piece of equipment, e.g., videoprocessor, still video recorder, etc.)
7. Staffed recovery area with electronic monitors, nurse call system, wall oxygen, and suction.
8. Refrigerator for clinical use.
9. Patient education room with printed and audiovisual materials and appropriate furnishings.
10. Radiologic facility within or adjacent to procedure unit.
11. Patient examination/consultation room(s).
12. Clean storage room for all endoscopes, accessories, and supplies and a medicine cabinet and locked narcotic cabinet.
13. Soiled utility room for cleaning and disinfection with exceptionally good ventilation (3,4), oversized sinks, ultrasonic cleaner, suction, and compressed air.

Medical Administration Area Organization and Equipment

The allotted space will depend on medical and nursing staffing patterns but should include the following:

1. Medical director's office furnished with video monitors wired to the procedure rooms.
2. Nursing office furnished with a computer for data entry and nurse call and intercom systems.
3. Staff physician office space with lab information and computer terminals, X-ray view boxes, dictating equipment, telephones, and intercom system.
4. Area(s) for photographic review and printing, and for computer report generation and printing.
5. Staff education room and library with video monitors, videocassette recorder (VCR), teaching videotapes, texts, and periodicals.
6. Staff changing rooms/bathrooms.
7. Conference room and lounge space with a refrigerator.

Receptionist Area Organization and Equipment

The receptionist area should be adjacent to the patient arrival and waiting area and readily accessible to the medical staff. Its size depends on the number of personnel, and space must be allotted for the following functions:

1. Patient identification imprinting equipment.
2. Computer terminals.
3. Filing and storage cabinets and racks for pertinent medical forms and supplies.
4. Patient record processing.
5. Telephones and intercom controls.
6. Incoming and outgoing mail sorters.
7. Patient education materials for mailing.

Secretarial Area Organization and Equipment

A computer-trained appointment secretary should be allotted separate adjacent space with a dedicated telephone number and computer equipment for generating and printing patient appointments. This secretary will also be responsible for patient log and cancellation records and the unit's pathology follow-up system.

Staff Responsibilities in the Procedure Unit

Medical

1. Consultation services to evaluate potential GI procedures.
2. Responsibility for medical management, patient care standards, ethical decisions, and procedural safety (5).
3. Active communication with nursing and secretarial staff.
4. Education of and responsibility for physicians in the training program.
5. Responsibility for documentation and follow-up of pathology reports and complication records.

Nursing

Nursing responsibilities in the procedure unit include competency in patient assessment, certain procedures [obtaining i.v. access, electronic monitoring, cardiopulmonary resuscitation (CPR) certification, etc.], verbal and written communication, and instrument care and handling. These competencies can be accomplished by well-supervised on-the-job experience; by attendance at training courses and seminars provided by regional chapters and the National Society for Gastrointestinal Nurses and Associates (SGNA); and by familiarization with texts, manuals (6), and journals related to the field. Membership in the SGNA is highly recommended, and certification by the organization should be encouraged.

Secretarial

The secretary-receptionists play pivotal roles in creating a comforting atmosphere and in fostering the smooth operation of the unit. They are the initial procedure unit contact for patients and are also responsible for coordinating their schedules. Their responsibilities include the following:

1. Maintain the schedule book. This requires knowledge of procedure time and room requirements as well as medical-nursing staffing patterns. In a busy referral hospital this is a complicated and most critical responsibility.
2. Provide imprinted medical forms for each patient, organize X-ray and laboratory data, and maintain patient files and procedure records.
3. Be familiar with computer-based and secretarial tasks.
4. Respond to institutional requirements for data and billing information.
5. Obtain some knowledge of medical insurance details (or know how to obtain it).
6. Make appointments and mail appropriate forms and information.
7. Arrange for patient transportation to and from unit.
8. Be alert to the needs of patients in the waiting area.
9. Label and deliver laboratory specimens.

Nursing Responsibilities to Patients

The staff's efforts toward patient education, comfort, and emotional support will help ensure a well-accepted and successfully administered procedure. The degree of patient preparation needed will depend on the type of procedure and the needs of the individual patient. All procedures require considerate, individualized attention to the patient by the staff. The following should be accomplished by the nursing staff (and/or the physician) (7,8):

1. Ascertain that all the preprocedure requirements have been met by the patient (e.g., nothing taken by mouth, bowel preparation completed, driver present or available).
2. Introduce yourself and explain your role in the procedure.
3. After chart review, assess through questioning, and with attention to verbal and nonverbal behavior, the patient's clinical status, including general health, allergies, and current medications. Note the patient's degree of apprehension and his or her ability to understand and communicate.
4. Assess the patient's understanding of the procedure.
5. Explain the procedure, in keeping with your assessment of the patient. Patients respond differently in anticipation of unfamiliar, potentially uncomfortable procedures. Some benefit from detailed explanations of what to expect, while others do not ask questions and express a desire to "get on with it and get it over with." The latter group of patients can become more agitated if too much effort is made to explain what they would rather not hear (9). In general, a description of the procedure including sensations likely to be experienced (such as numbness of the throat, a brief needle stick, abdominal cramps) is more valuable than detailed scientific explanations (10). The need for the test, alternative therapy, and possible risks and complications should be presented in a straightforward manner by the physician. Detailed descriptions of all complications are not necessary (11). It is helpful to have available a variety of adjunctive audiovisual materials, including printed patient guides, videotapes, and audio slide equipment, to be offered to the patient when he or she is confronted with the need for a certain study, and again just prior to the procedure.
6. Assess the patient's understanding of your explanation, and allow sufficient time for questions.
7. Review discharge instructions prior to conscious sedation.

8. Witness granting of informed consent.
9. Perform the needed preparation [vital signs, i.v. access, and if necessary, draw blood samples, administer prophylactic antibiotics for subacute bacterial endocarditis (SBE), etc.]
10. Using your judgment, administer topical anesthesia i.v. sedation, and other medication as per physician's orders, (12, 13).
11. During the procedure, monitor the patient's clinical condition (change in vital signs, need for more medication, possible complications), and provide support and reassurance to the patient.
12. At the end of the procedure and when determining readiness for discharge, reassess the patient's clinical status (vital signs, mentation, physical complaints, etc.). Review written postprocedural instructions (possible aftereffects and complications, medication schedules, return appointment date) with the patient and family member if possible, obtain signature, and provide patient with a copy.
13. Accurately document patient care, responses, and medications on appropriate medical chart forms (14).
14. Make appropriate patient referrals to Social Work, Home Health, Nutritionist, etc.

Equipment- and Unit-Related Responsibilities

1. Adherence to universal blood and body fluid precautions (all personnel) and appropriate inspection, cleaning, and disinfection of all equipment and accessories immediately after each procedure according to infection control guidelines and manufacturers' standards (15–18).
2. Maintain an appropriate inventory of all equipment and accessories.
3. Coordinate patient flow and schedule changes with the secretary and involved physicians.
4. Provide and maintain written care standards, unit policies, and procedure and job descriptions to ensure continuity in the unit for institutional accountability.
5. Maintain instrument repair records for in-service education and purchase decisions.

6. Maintain an error-proof system for handling biological specimens and for pathology report follow-up.
7. Order and distribute unit supplies, equipment, medications, and linens.
8. Provide in-service education programs.
9. Document adherence to all applicable Joint Commission on Accreditation of Healthcare Organizations (JCAHO) standards.
10. Maintain equipment and accessory inventory records.
11. Uphold cost-containment measures.
12. Involve yourself with and document quality assessment activities (19).

In conclusion, with the rapid growth of diagnostic and therapeutic procedures in gastroenterology, the goals of safe, efficient, cost-effective, and considerate patient care can best be met by having a well-trained staff, sufficient space and equipment, open lines of communication, realistic scheduling, and standardized procedural practices where possible.

REFERENCES

1. Sivak MV Jr, Senick JM (1987): The endoscopy unit. *Gastroenterologic Endoscopy*. Philadelphia: WB Saunders Co.
2. Society of Gastrointestinal Nurses and Associates (SGNA) (Jan 1991): *Manipulation of Endoscopes During Endoscopic Procedures by Gastroenterology Nurses and Associates*, pp 1–2. SGNA Position Statement. Society of Gastrointestinal Nurses and Associates, Rochester, New York.
3. Rutala WA, Hamory BH (1989): Expanding role of hospital epidemiology: employee health-chemical exposure in the health care setting. *Infect Control Hosp Epidemiol* 10:261–266.
4. Wiggins P, McCurdy SA, Zeidenberg W (1989): Epistaxis due to glutaraldehyde exposure. *J Occup Med* 31:854–856.
5. Vilardell F (1980): Ethical problems in the management of gastrointestinal patients. *Endoscopy* (Suppl):1–12.
6. Hardick M (1989): *Manual of Gastrointestinal Procedures*, 2nd ed. Society of Gastrointestinal Nurses and Associates, Rochester, New York.
7. Standards of Training and Practice Committee, American Society for Gastrointestinal Endoscopy (1988): *Standards of Practice of Gastrointestinal Endoscopy, Supplement*, p 88. American Society for Gastrointestinal Endoscopy, Boston.

8. Practice Committee, Society of Gastrointestinal Nurses and Associates (SGNA) (1991): *Standards for Practice in the Endoscopy Setting.* SGNA Monograph Series. Wilson-Cook Medical, Inc., Winston-Salem.

9. Shipley RH, Butt JH, Farbry JE, Horwitz B (1977): Psychological preparation for endoscopy: physiological and behavioral changes in patients with differing coping styles for stress. *Gastrointest Endosc* 24:9–13.

10. Hartfield MD, Cason CL (1981): Effective information on emotional responses during the barium enema. *Nurs Res* 30:151–155.

11. Roling GT, Pressgrove LW, Keefe EB, Raffin SB (1977): An appraisal of patient's reactions to "informed consent" for peroral endoscopy. *Gastrointest Endosc* 24:69–70.

12. Society of Gastrointestinal Nurses and Associates (SGNA) Board of Directors (Jan 1991): *Responsibilities of the Gastroenterology Registered Nurse Related to Conscious Sedation*, pp 1–2. SGNA Position Statement. Society of Gastrointestinal Nurses and Associates, Rochester, New York.

13. Fleischer D (1990): Sedation and monitoring during gastrointestinal endoscopy. *Gastrointest Endosc* 36(Suppl.):S2–S22.

14. Bodinsky G, Falconio M (May 1989): *Documentation: Charting to Standardize*, pp 1–4. SGNA Monograph Series. Society of Gastrointestinal Nurses and Associates, Rochester, New York.

15. Practice Committee, Society of Gastrointestinal Nurses and Associates (SGNA) (1990): *Recommended Guidelines for Infection Control in Gastrointestinal Endoscopy Settings.* SGNA Monograph Series. Wilson-Cook Medical, Inc., Winston-Salem.

16. Standards of Training and Practice Committee, American Society for Gastrointestinal Endoscopy (1988): *Infection Control During Gastrointestinal Endoscopy.* Boston.

17. Schaffner M (1990): Infection control issues in the gastrointestinal endoscopy unit. *Gastroenterol Nurs* 12(4):279–284.

18. Gorse GJ, Messner RL (1991): Infection control practices in gastrointestinal endoscopy in the United States: a national survey. *Gastroenterol Nurs* 14(2):72–79.

19. Practice Committee, Society of Gastrointestinal Nurses and Associates (SGNA) (1990): *Quality Assurance for the Endoscopy Department.* SGNA Monograph Series. Wilson-Cook Medical, Inc., Winston-Salem.

1 / Oral and Nasal Gastrointestinal Intubation

Meredith P. Reinhold and C. Thomas Nuzum

There is an increasing variety of gastrointestinal tubes available. The type of tube selected is determined by its intended use, efficacy, and cost-effectiveness. Due to their tendency to stiffen with time (1) and to produce tissue irritation or necrosis, polyvinyl-chloride tubes should generally be relegated to decompression and drainage, gastric lavage, and diagnostic sampling. Pliable small-bore silicone or polyurethane tubes are best for long-term infusion. In addition, silicone tubes may produce less patient discomfort (2), but reduced clogging and enhanced feeding flow have been reported with polyurethane tubes (1). Large-bore orogastric tubes are most effective for removing clots (3).

Indicated below are general features of oral and nasogastric tubes, followed by specific details for each type of tube:

General Indications

1. Gastric lavage.
2. Gastrointestinal feeding and medication administration.
3. Gastrointestinal decompression.
4. Gastrointestinal diagnostic sampling and testing.

General Contraindications

1. Nasopharyngeal or upper esophageal obstruction.
2. Severe maxillofacial trauma and/or basilar skull fracture.
3. Severe uncontrolled coagulopathy.
4. Varices and severe esophagitis are contraindications to pro-

longed use of large-bore polyvinylchloride tubes. More pliable, small-diameter tubes reduce trauma but do not abolish the drawing of acid upstream along the exterior surface of the tube ("wick effect").
5. Bullous disorders of the esophageal mucosa.

General Complications
During Intubation

1. Nasal or pharyngeal trauma.
2. Laryngeal trauma.
3. Laryngotracheal obstruction.
4. Nasotracheal intubation or transbronchial perforation (4–6).
5. Esophageal or gastric trauma or perforation (7).
6. Intracranial penetration (8,9).

During Use

1. Pulmonary aspiration (10,11).
2. Gastroesophageal reflux.
3. Mucosal injury and ulceration (12).
4. Chronic irritation causing rhinitis, sinusitis (13,14), pharyngitis, otitis media (15), and rarely, vocal cord paralysis (16).

During Extubation

1. Mucosal damage.
2. Entrapment (17–20).

General Patient Preparation

1. Give nothing by mouth for several hours.
2. Explain procedure to patient, including route, purpose, and anticipated duration of intubation.
3. Have the patient sit upright, or raise the head of the bed. If this is not possible, passing the tube with the patient in the

left lateral decubitus position has less risk of aspiration than if the patient is supine.

4. Check for nasal obstruction. Have the patient inhale briskly through each nostril and use the more patent nostril for intubation.

5. Test the gag reflex. Patients unable to gag are at increased risk of pulmonary aspiration. Local anesthesia is indicated only for the most difficult cases.

General Equipment

1. Gastrointestinal tube of choice.
2. Water-soluble lubricant.
3. Cup of water and straw.
4. Emesis basin and towel.
5. Tongue blade and flashlight.
6. Aspirating and irrigating syringes.
7. Tincture of benzoin, scissors, and tape or semipermeable transparent membrane dressing.
8. Stethoscope.

Specific Tubes

Styleted Feeding Tubes (e.g., Entriflex, Corpak)

Characteristics

1. These are long silicone or polyurethane tubes, 36 to 43 in. in length. Transpyloric feedings require 43-in. tubes, but they can be used for gastric feeding when passed to the shorter length.
2. Intraluminal diameter of 5 to 12 French.
3. Distal tip weighted by a tungsten bolus.
4. Placement stylet packaged with tubes.
5. Delivery ports encased in nonperforable material for safer reuse of stylet, when necessary.
6. Radiopaque markings to aid in fluoroscopic placement.
7. Increased pliability, to reduce tissue irritation and increase taping options to the face.

Special Indications

1. Inability or unwillingness to ingest sufficient nutrients and/or prescribed medications.
2. Impaired swallowing or gastric emptying.
3. Transition from parenteral to oral alimentation or adjunctive use with limited oral feeding.
4. To reduce (but not eliminate) pancreatic or biliary stimulation.

Specific Contraindications

1. Complete gastric or intestinal obstruction.
2. Severe gastroesophageal reflux.
3. Ileus.
4. Patient intolerance to tube.
5. Intractable vomiting.
6. Impaired cough and gag reflexes, and mental status changes are relative contraindications.

Specific Preparation

1. Read package insert and retain in the patient's chart.
2. Have fluoroscopy available.

Equipment

See also General Equipment

1. Small-bore feeding tube and stylet.
2. 3-cc Syringe for aspirating.
3. Water and 10-cc syringe to activate hydromer lubricant.
4. Liquid silicone lubricant.
5. pH testing supplies.
6. Contrast material and metoclopramide.

Procedure for Direct Placement

1. Estimate length of tube to be inserted. For 90% confidence of placing the tip 1 to 10 cm beyond the cardia in adults, use

Hanson's formula (21): (NEX − 50)/2 + 50 cm. Mark the tube 50 cm from its tip. Then, with the patient's head in a neutral position, hold the tip of the tube on the patient's nose and lay the tube along the shortest path from the nose (N) to the earlobe (E) to the xyphoid (X) process. Mark the tube where it reaches the end of the xyphoid. The length of insertion should be halfway between 50 cm and the xyphoid mark. Conventional insertion to the NEX distance placed more than 10 cm of tube in 26% of subjects studied. Unless it traverses the pyloris, excess tube in the stomach often loops, pushing the tip into the fundus or cardia.

2. Lubricate tube or activate hydromer lubricant, and examine tube for rough edges or blocked holes. The tube should be emptied of any liquid that might trickle into the trachea. Fix stylet in place, if packaged separately. In more distal placements, removal of the stylet is easier when it has been lubricated with liquid silicone.

3. With the patient's head tilted down, gently push the tube through the nares, aiming it back and then down to conform with the nasopharynx. If pointed too high, the tip will abrade the turbinates.

4. As the tip reaches the posterior pharyngeal wall, have the patient sip water through a straw or initiate dry swallows. This is the most uncomfortable part of the procedure. If resistance is met, retract and try again. Do not force the tube. If the patient coughs or is unable to speak, the tube may be in the trachea. However, smaller tubes do not always elicit these signs. In the unconscious patient, cyanosis may be the first sign of tracheal intubation.

5. Pass the tube to the predetermined length, checking that it is not coiled in the patient's pharynx and mouth. Remove stylet slowly with slightly jiggling motion to reduce adherence to the lumen.

6. Confirm the tube's placement in the stomach by gently aspirating gastric contents with a 3-cc syringe, and check the pH (22). Verifying tube position by auscultation alone is not as helpful since the sounds of air in the bronchial tree can be mistaken for gastric insufflation (23). We also recommend radiologic verification if other methods of verification have

failed. This is mandatory in the anesthetized or comatose patient.

7. After applying tincture of benzoin, tape tube to nose and/or cheek. First, cut 1½ × 1-in. piece of nonallergenic tape or semipermeable transparent membrane dressing material (which reduces visual distraction). Then, split one end in half and place the uncut end on the patient's nose, wrapping the cut ends around tube. Be careful to minimize tube contact with the nostril.

8. If small-bowel placement is desired, after gastric placement is verified, place the patient on his or her right side for several hours. Maintain 20 to 30 cm of tube slack between the taping location on the cheek and the nares, in order to allow further passage of the tube into the duodenum.

9. When the slack has disappeared, have the patient lie on his or her back, and then on the left side to promote the tube's passage into the jejunum. Secure the tube to the nose.

10. Check the tube position fluoroscopically. If it has not passed through the pylorus, give metoclopramide, 10 mg i.v., and recheck fluoroscopically several minutes later. If it is difficult to determine the position, instill a small amount of dilute contrast material. Irrigate with water after using contrast material to avoid clogging.

Procedure for Endoscopically Guided Placement (24,25)

Endoscopically guided placement is possible in the presence of esophageal diverticula, strictures, tortuosity, and obstructing lesions. This method is also useful for transpyloric placement in the presence of surgical alterations, gastroparesis, and pyloric obstruction.

1. Tie a small loop of umbilical tape to the distal tip of the tube.
2. Pass the endoscope into the esophagus.
3. Pass the lubricated, styleted feeding tube alongside the endoscope until the loop is visible.
4. Pass grasping forceps through the endoscope and grasp the loop. Guide the feeding tube to the appropriate position.

5. Keep the stylet in place until the endoscope is removed. This prevents displacement of the tube by friction.
6. Confirm tube placement fluoroscopically.
7. Remove the stylet with a gentle jiggling motion.

Procedure for Endoscopically Placed Guide Wire Replacement (e.g., Endo-Tube)

This method can be successful in the presence of strictured or edematous gut through which an endoscope cannot pass. Its disadvantage is the diameter of the stainless-steel weighted tip which must be passed through the nostril over the guide wire.

1. Perform endoscopy to the second or third position of the duodenum if possible.
2. Using fluoroscopic guidance, place the guide wire through the endoscope, to the desired location.
3. With fluoroscopic guidance, remove the endoscope while feeding the guide wire through the channel to maintain placement.
4. Using the 8 French polyurethane cannula provided, transfer the guide wire from the oral to a nasal exit. Remove slack and fluoroscopically check the position.
5. Remove the cannula.
6. Activate the hydromer lubricant by flushing the feeding tube with 20 cc of water.
7. Using fluoroscopic control, pass the feeding tube over the guide wire.
8. Recheck the placement fluoroscopically before feeding.

Special Complications

1. Vomiting or aspiration due to displacement of the tube from the small bowel to the stomach, or from the stomach to the esophagus.
2. Perforation of the gut because of misuse or reuse of the stylet or as a result of overzealous use of the stylet to unclog the tube.

3. Clogging of the tube due to inadequate irrigation or improper medication instillation techniques (26–28).
4. Tube rupture as a result of too much irrigation pressure, or the use of an irrigating syringe smaller than 50 cc in size.

Gastric Decompression Tubes
(e.g., Salem Sump Tube)
Characteristics

1. Polyvinylchloride tubes 43 to 48 in. long in 12, 14, 16, and 18 French diameter (also in pediatric sizes).
2. Double lumen to maintain atmospheric pressure for adequate drainage and to reduce adherence to the mucosa.
3. Radiopaque sentinel line and periodic markings.

Specific Indications

1. Decompression due to gastric atony, ileus, or bowel obstruction.

Specific Contraindications

See General Contraindications.

Specific Preparation

See General Patient Preparation.

Equipment

See General Equipment.

Specific Procedure

1. Soften the polyvinylchloride tube in warm water before passing it.

2. Place the tube in the same manner as for feeding tubes except that no stylet is needed.
3. Tube position can be verified by aspiration of gastric contents.

Specific Complications

1. Clogging of either or both lumens due to inadequate irrigation.
2. Loss of patency of small lumen due to crushing by a clamp.
3. Tissue damage due to improper taping at nostril.

Gastric Lavage Tubes (*e.g.*, Edlich, Ewald)
Characteristics

1. Polyvinylchloride or rubber tubes 36 in. long with 34 French diameter.
2. Large ports.

Specific Indications

1. To empty the esophagus or stomach of particulate material (e.g., soft bezoars).
2. To irrigate blood clots, toxins, or other substances requiring large-volume lavage.

Specific Contraindications

See General Contraindications.

Specific Preparation

See General Patient Preparation.

1. Soften polyvinyl lavage tube in warm water.
2. Drain all water from tube.

Equipment

See General Equipment.
1. Overbed table for two large basins.
2. Water-resistant covering for the patient's upper body.
3. Extra-large lavage syringe. (Save, wash, and disinfect as per endoscopic equipment.)
4. Clamp. (Large hemostats are more effective than the sliding clamp which is provided.)

Specific Procedure

1. Pass the well-lubricated tube orally with the head partially flexed after initial placement beyond the hypopharynx.
2. Check position by aspiration and auscultation before initiating lavage.
3. Keep the patient warm if an iced lavage solution is used.

Specific Complications

1. Mucosal trauma during insertion or during removal if suction is not released.
2. Aspiration if tube is not clamped during removal.

Intestinal Decompression Tubes (29,30)
Characteristics

1. Cantor tube: 10 ft long, 16 French diameter, siliconized, radiopaque, single lumen with balloon to hold mercury.
2. Miller-Abbott: 10 ft long, 16 French diameter, red rubber, double lumen with balloon to hold mercury.

Specific Indications

1. To decompress the small bowel.

Specific Contraindications

See General Contraindications.

1. Small-bowel obstruction.

Specific Preparation

See General Patient Preparation.

Equipment

See General Equipment.

1. 5 to 9 ml of mercury (5 ml for patients with active peristalsis and 7 to 9 ml for those with an ileus and absent bowel sounds).
2. No. 21 gauge needle and 10-cc syringe.
3. Umbilical tape to form support loop for the tube.
4. Basin of hot water for Cantor tube.

Specific Procedures

1. Read the package insert and retain in the patient's chart.
2. Do not affix the tube to the nostril until full passage is achieved.
3. Advance the tube according to package insert instructions.
4. Deflate Miller-Abbott tube before removal.

Specific Complications

1. Knotting of the tube in the stomach due to too rapid passage.
2. Failure to reach desired location due to obstruction or motility disorder.
3. Tissue damage or necrosis due to lack of slack during passage.
4. Rare: Passage through the anus of the mercury bolus. If this occurs, cut off bolus section of tube and remove the tube according to instructions.
   Caution: Adhere to institutional requirements for disposal of mercury.

Short-Term Use Tubes (e.g., Bardic, Levin)

Characteristics

1. Polyvinylchloride tubes, generally come in 42- to 50-in. lengths with a variety of French diameters.
2. Single-lumen tube without radiopaque markings.
3. Least expensive, thus suited to short-term use.

Specific Indications

1. Diagnostic sampling [pH, presence of blood (31)].
2. Adaptive uses, such as Bernstein and saline load tests.
3. Installation of balanced electrolyte solution in whole-gut lavage.

REFERENCES

1. Petrosino BM, Christian BJ, Wolfe J, Becker H (1989): Implications of selected problems with naso-enteral tube feedings. *Crit Care Nurs Q* 12(3):1–18.
2. Herrman ME, Lyehr RM, Tanhoefner H, Emde C, Richen EO (1989): Subjective distress during continuous enteral alimentation: superiority of silicone rubber to polyurethane. *JPEN* 13:281–285.
3. Peterson WL (1983): Gastrointestinal bleeding. In: *Gastrointestinal Disease*, edited by MH Sleisenger, JS Fordtran, p 181. WB Saunders Company, Philadelphia.
4. Wendell GD, Lenchner GS, Promisloff RA (1991): Pneumothorax complicating small small-bore feeding tube placement. *Arch Intern Med* 151:599–602.
5. Harris MR, Huseby JS (1989): Pulmonary complications from vasoenteral feeding tube insertion in an intensive care unit: incidence and prevention. *Crit Care Med* 17:917–919.
6. Carey TS, Holcombe BJ (1991): Endotrachial intubation as a risk factor for complications of nasoenteric tube insertion. *Crit Care Med* 19:427–429.
7. Jackson RH, Payne DK, Bacon BR (1990): Esophageal perforation due to naso-gastric intubation. *Am J Gastroenterol* 85:439–442.
8. Koch KJ, Becker GJ, Edwards MK, Hoover RL (1989): Intracranial placement of a naso-gastric tube. *AJNR* 10(2):443–444.
9. Glasser SA, Garfinkle W, Scanlon M (1990): Intracranial complications during insertion of a naso/gastric tube. *AJNR* 11:1170.

10. Murphy LM (1991): Incidence of pulmonary aspiration in intubated patients receiving enteral nutrition through wide- and narrow-bore nasogastric feeding tubes. Letter. *Heart Lung* 20:426–427.

11. Sands JA (1991): Incidents of pulmonary aspiration in intubated patients receiving enteral nutrition through wide- and narrow-bore naso-gastric feeding tubes. *Heart Lung* 20:75–80.

12. Rombeau JL, Miller RA (1979): *Nasoenteric Tube Feeding; Practical Aspects*, p 10. Hedeco, Mt. View, California.

13. Desmond P, Raman R, Idikula J (1991): Effect of naso-gastric tubes on the nose and maxillary sinus. *Crit Care Med* 19:509–511.

14. Bos AP, Tibboel D, Hazebroek PW, Hoeve H, Meradji M, Molenaar JC (1989): Sinusitis: hidden source of sepsis in post-operative pediatric intensive care patients. *Crit Care Med* 17:886–888.

15. Wake M, McCullough DE, Binnington JD (1990): Effect of naso-gastric on eustachian tube function. *J Laryngol Otol* 104:17–19.

16. Sofferman RA, Haisch CE, Kirchener JA, Hardin NJ (1990): The naso/gastric tube syndrome. *Laryngoscope* 100:962–968.

17. Sliwa JA, Marciniak C (1989): A complication of naso/gastric tube removal. *Arch Phys Med Rehabil* 70:702–704.

18. Urschel JD, Stockburger HJ (1990): Endoscopic extraction of an entrapped naso/gastric tube. *Am Surg* 56:730–732.

19. Jones M (1989): The knotted naso/gastric tube: a simple solution. *Br J Clin Pract*. 43:183–184.

20. Thomson HG (1989): "Granny's knot" as a complication of naso/gastric tube feeding(N). *Ear Nose Throat J* 68:636.

21. Hanson RL (1979): Predictive criteria for length of naso/gastric tube insertion for tube feeding. *JPEN* 3:160–163.

22. Metheny N, Williams P, Wiersema L, Luehrle MA, Eisenberg P, McSweeney M (1989): Effectiveness of pH measurements in predicting feeding tube placement. *Nurs Res* 38:280–285.

23. Metheny N, McSweeney M, Wehrle MA, Wiesema L (1990): Effectiveness of the auscultatory method in predicting feeding tube location. *Nurs Res* 39:262–267.

24. Stark SP, Sharpe JN, Larson GM (1991): Endoscopically placed naso-enteral feeding tubes. Indications and techniques. *Am Surg* 57:203–205.

25. Rives DA, LeRoy JL, Hawkins ML, Bowden TA Jr (1989): Endoscopically assisted naso/jejunal feeding tube placement. *Am Surg* 55:88–91.

26. Benson DW, Griggs BA, Hamilton F, Hiyama DT, Bower RH (1990): Clogging of feeding tubes: a randomized trial of a newly designed tube. *Nutr Clin Pract* 5:107–110.

27. Bommarito AA, Heinzelmann MJ, Boysen DA (1989): A new approach to the management of obstructed enteral feeding tubes. *Nutr Clin Pract* 4:111–114.

28. Marcuard SP, Stegall KS (1990): Unclogging feeding tubes with pancreatic enzyme. *JPEN* 14:198–200.
29. Snyder CL, Ferrell KL, Goodale RL, Leonard AS (1990): Nonoperative management of small-bowel obstruction with endoscopic long intestinal tube placement. *Am Surg* 56:587–592.
30. Terasaka R, Itoh H, Nakafusa Y, Matsuo K (1990): Effectiveness of a long intestinal tube in a 1-stage operation for obstructing carcinoma of the left colon. *Dis Colon Rectum* 33:245–248.
31. Cuellar RE, Gavaler JS, Alexander JA, et al (1990): Gastrointestinal tract hemorrhage. The value of a naso/gastric aspirate. *Arch Intern Med* 150:1381–1384.

2 / The Saline Load Test

C. Thomas Nuzum

Gastric emptying is assessed by physical exam (succession splash), radiography, radioisotope scanning, and intubation studies measuring gastric contents. The saline load test (1) lacks the accuracy, precision, and physiological relevance of infusions employing unabsorbed markers (2), but merits description because of common clinical use.

Indications

1. To test for impaired gastric emptying.
2. To assess healing, efficacy of treatment, and readiness for dietary advancement in patients known to have gastric outlet obstruction and/or disorders of motility.

Contraindications

1. See contraindications to nasogastric intubation (chapter by Reinhold and Nuzum).
2. Small obstructed gastric pouch or voluminous gastroesophageal reflux.
3. Diseases managed by stringent salt and fluid restriction. Water is not substituted for saline because hypotonic duodenal fluid retards gastric emptying (3).

Preparation

1. Nothing by mouth for at least 4 hr.
2. Explain procedure to patient.

Equipment

1. No. 16 French polyvinyl tube with usual accessories for naso-gastric intubation (see chapter by Reinhold and Nuzum), including "catheter-tipped" 50-cc syringes.
2. Sodium chloride, 750 ml 0.9%, in an open vessel or i.v. infusion set.

Procedure

1. Place the nasogastric tube (see chapter by Reinhold and Nuzum).
2. Confirm the tube position radiographically.
3. Aspirate any gastric fluid.
4. Place the patient supine (as originally described) (1) or in left lateral position.
5. Infuse 750 ml saline in less than 5 min from an i.v. set or via syringes.
6. At 30 min, quickly aspirate the gastric contents completely. Obtain as much fluid as possible in the left lateral decubitus, supine, right lateral decubitus, and upright positions. At each position, move the tube in and out over a ± 5-cm range.
7. Measure total volume withdrawn in step 6, i.e., the saline residue.

Interpretation

Goldstein and Boyle (1) performed saline load tests in 23 adult men with clinical evidence of gastric retention due to duodenal ulcer (except for two antral cancers) and in 69 control subjects (Table 1). On retesting after 24 hr of suction and fluid/electrolyte replacement, 15 of their 23 patients improved, suggesting a reversible component of the obstruction. The authors concluded that "if the initial saline residue is 400 ml or more, it may be said with some confidence that the patient has clinical gastric retention. Values between 300 and 400 ml are suggestive of gastric retention."

The saline load test is not specific for obstruction. Without a marker it fails to distinguish the "retention" of pyloric stenosis

TABLE 1. Original Saline Load Test Results (1)

		Patients (23)	
Control Subjects (69)		Untreated (20)	8–10 hr Nasogastric Suction (3)
Mean residue (ml)	60	640	290
Range (ml)	<200 (63)	370–750	280–295
	205–385 (6)		

from the hypersecretion of Zollinger-Ellison syndrome. Retention occurs in many motility disturbances, but because the stomach's emptying rates differ for solid and liquid phases (4,5), a normal liquid residual volume does not rule out disorders like diabetic gastroparesis. The saline load test is of value insofar as it is sensitive to obstruction, simple to perform at the bedside, and cheap. It can show the severity of an obstruction underestimated by conventional radiography and endoscopy (6). A symposium addresses in detail the methodology and interpretation of other gastric-emptying tests (7).

REFERENCES

1. Goldstein H, Boyle JD (1965): The saline load test—a bedside evaluation of gastric retention. *Gastroenterology* 49:375–380.
2. Hunt JN, Knox MT (1968): Regulation of gastric emptying. In: *Handbook of Physiology*, Sect 6, Vol IV, edited by CF Code, pp 1917–1935. American Physiological Society, Washington, DC.
3. Mecroff JC, Go VLW, Philips SF (1975): Control of gastric emptying by osmolality of duodenal contents in man. *Gastroenterology* 68:1144–1151.
4. Pelot D, Dana ER, Berk JE, Dixon G (1972): Comparative assessment of gastric emptying by the "barium-burger" and saline load tests. *Am J Gastroenterol* 58:411–416.
5. Rees WDW, Miller LJ, Malagelada J-R (1980): Dyspepsia, antral motor dysfunction, and gastric stasis of solids. *Gastroenterology* 78:360–365.
6. Caldwell JH, Cerilli GJ (1977): Adult hypertrophic pyloric stenosis. Report of an unusual case detected by saline load test. *Am J Gastroenterol* 67:261–264.
7. Dubois A, Castell DO, eds (1984): *Esophageal and Gastric Emptying*. CRC Press, Boca Raton.

3 / Insertion of the Minnesota Tube

Kim L. Isaacs and Sidney L. Levinson

The Minnesota four lumen esophagogastric tamponade tube is used in the treatment of hemorrhage from varices in the esophagus and stomach (1) (Fig. 1). This tube is a modification of the widely used, three-lumen Sengstaken-Blakemore tube which incorporates an internal separate esophageal suction port to the existing gastric suction port, gastric balloon, and esophageal balloon lumens (2,3). The Linton-Nachlas tube also has an esophageal suction port but lacks the esophageal balloon. The Minnesota tube has been demonstrated to be fairly well tolerated by patients. Its design may help to prevent aspiration of esophageal contents (1).

The Minnesota tube is used for control of hemorrhage from esophageal varices, documented by endoscopy or in rare cases angiography, which continue to bleed despite aggressive medical management including lavage, correction of blood-clotting abnormalities, intravenous vasopressin or somatostatin infusion, and acute sclerotherapy (4). An alternative approach, currently under investigation, is the use of a transjugular intrahepatic portasystemic shunt for uncontrollable bleeding.

Indication

Acute bleeding from esophageal or gastric varices unresponsive to medical therapy including emergent sclerotherapy.

Contraindications
Absolute

1. Patients in whom variceal bleeding has stopped.

27

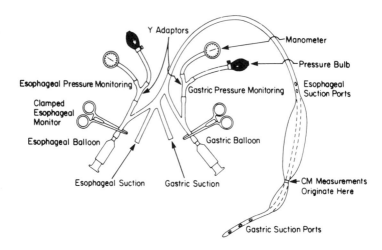

FIG. 1. Minnesota four-lumen tube.

2. Patients with recent surgery involving the esophagogastric junction.
3. Patients with known esophageal stricture.

Relative

1. Poorly informed support staff (5).
2. Improper equipment (defective tube, no traction helmet).
3. Congestive heart failure.
4. Respiratory failure.
5. Cardiac arrhythmias.
6. Hiatal hernia.
7. Incomplete lavage.
8. Inability to demonstrate a variceal source of bleeding.
9. Recurrent bleeding after initial successful tamponade in an operative or sclerotherapy candidate (6,7).
10. Esophageal ulceration (secondary to reflux esophagitis or previous sclerotherapy—in these cases, the gastric balloon may be used but not the esophageal balloon).

Preparation

1. Perform endoscopy to confirm the source of bleeding and attempt sclerotherapy as a primary mode of treating acute variceal bleeding.
2. Protect airway and consider intubation in selected patients.
3. Transfuse as necessary for resuscitation and to improve coagulation abnormalities.
4. Anesthetize the oropharynx.
5. With the patient on the left side in semi-Fowler's position, lavage stomach with tap water using an adult gastric lavage or other large-bore tube.
6. Test the balloons by insufflating each with air and examining for leaks under water.
7. Connect a mercury manometer to the gastric balloon and inflate with 100-cc increments of air to 500 cc, recording manometric pressure at each point.
8. Instruct the staff caring for the patient in the use of the tube, complications that may arise, and measures for emergency removal.

Equipment

A commercially available four-lumen tube with aspiration ports in the gastric and esophageal sections, a spherical gastric balloon capable of holding 500 cc air, and a sausage-shaped esophageal balloon with reinforced rubber proximally attached to the gastric balloon. There are ports available for insufflation of esophageal and gastric balloons and for pressure monitoring of both of these balloons.

Other Equipment

1. Topical anesthesia and tongue blades or swabs.
2. Two wall-suction setups with plastic connectors to adapt gastric and esophageal ports to suction tubing.
3. Rubber- or adhesive tape–shod clamps for gastric and esophageal balloon ports.

4. Two manometers with pressure bulbs attached by connector to one port of the gastric balloon lumen and one port of the esophageal balloon lumen.
5. Water-soluble lubricant.
6. Catheter (60 cc)-tipped syringes.
7. Football helmet or catcher's mask to secure the tube to one in place. An over-the-bed traction can be used but this markedly limits the mobility of the patient.
8. Adhesive tape.
9. Scissors, which should be taped to the top of the bed or to the top of the helmet.

Procedure

1. Suction all air from the balloons and insert plastic plugs.
2. Clamp rubber-shod clamps on the two pressure-monitoring outlets.
3. Lubricate the tube and pass it through the patient's mouth until the 45-cm mark is located past the dentate ridge. Do not pass the tube through the nares unless orogastric passage is impossible (increased risk of necrosis of the nasal septum, sinusitis). The 45-cm mark is measured from the junction of the esophageal and gastric balloons. This should be taken into consideration in patients who are status post esophageal or gastric surgery. If blind passage is not possible, endoscopically place a guide wire, then pass the Minnesota tube with the tip cut off over the guide wire (8). Confirm the position of the tube fluoroscopically so the tip is below the diaphragm.
4. Apply suction to the gastric and esophageal ports.
5. Remove the rubber-shod clamp and plastic plug from the gastric ports. Check the connection of the gastric pressure-monitoring outlet to the mercury manometer. Use the catheter-tip syringe to introduce 100 cc air increments through the gastric insufflation port. Check the manometer readings for correlation with preintubation readings. If the intragastric balloon pressure after intubation is 15 mm Hg greater than that which was produced prior to the intubation, then the balloon should be deflated, as it may be located in the esoph-

agus. Deflate the balloon immediately if the patient experiences chest pain.

6. When the gastric balloon is inflated with 450 to 500 cc air, clamp the air inlet and pressure-monitoring outlets and pull the tube back gently until resistance is felt against the gastroesophageal junction.

7. With a minimum of tension on the tube, fix the upper end of the tube as it exits from the mouth to the crossbar of a football helmet or a catcher's mask. Over-the-bed traction with a 1-lb weight may be used, but it is difficult to maintain proper position and allows much less patient mobility (9).

8. Observe the nature of the drainage from the gastric and esophageal ports. If bleeding persists from either port, inflate the esophageal balloon. To do this, first check the connection between the esophageal pressure-monitoring port and the manometer, then inflate to a pressure of 25 to 45 mm Hg, using the lowest pressure needed to stop bleeding through both the gastric and esophageal ports. Never inflate the esophageal balloon before the gastric balloon. Double clamp the tube. Periodically check the balloon pressure with the mercury manometer or keep the manometer attached for constant monitoring.

9. Elevate the head of the bed 6 to 10 in. Tape the scissors to the helmet or the head of the bed for quick access in case the balloons need immediate deflation.

Postprocedure

1. Verify the tube position by stat portable X-ray (7).

2. After bleeding has been controlled, reduce the pressure in the esophageal balloon 5 mm Hg every 3 hr until 25 mm Hg is reached without bleeding. Due to the risk of esophageal pressure necrosis, deflation of the esophageal balloon is performed for 5 min every 6 hr.

3. Manually check the tube tension at 3-hr intervals. Do not manipulate the tube unnecessarily.

4. Give nothing by mouth. Institute oral hygiene. If necessary, give medications through the gastric port.

5. Check both the gastric and esophageal return regularly and

flush both lumens if there is any question of clogging. Barium should never be instilled through the tube, since impaction of balloons could occur, requiring surgical removal of the tube (10).

6. If respiratory distress occurs due to proximal migration of the esophageal balloon with occlusion of the airway, the tube must be removed immediately! *Grasp the tube at the mouth, transect with scissors above the grasping hand but below the entrance of the three channel inlets, and pull out the tube.*

7. If hemostasis persists for 24 hr, deflate the esophageal balloon. If there is no recurrence of bleeding over the next 6 to 12 hr, deflate the gastric balloon and release tension but leave the Minnesota tube in place. If bleeding recurs, the gastric balloon and, if necessary, the esophageal balloon may be reinflated for an additional 24 hr (Fig. 2).

8. In the case of rebleeding, alternatives such as sclerotherapy and surgery should be reconsidered as there is a high mortality rate among patients who rebleed (6).

9. If bleeding does not recur by 24 hr after deflation, remove the Minnesota tube and transect it to ensure that it will not be reused. Removal is best done when there is adequate staff available to manage any rebleeding that might occur.

Complications

Major

1. Aspiration. In older series, this was a significant cause of death (7). The greatest risk for aspiration occurs during insertion. Airway protection with intubation should be strongly considered in selected patients (11).

2. Airway occlusion secondary to proximal migration of the tube. This is usually secondary to deflation of the gastric balloon while the esophageal balloon remains inflated (5).

3. Pressure effects. Rupture of the esophagus, laceration or ulceration of the stomach, and pressure necrosis of the hypopharynx or alae nasi may occur with prolonged balloon inflation or excessive pressures. Rupture of the esophagus is a

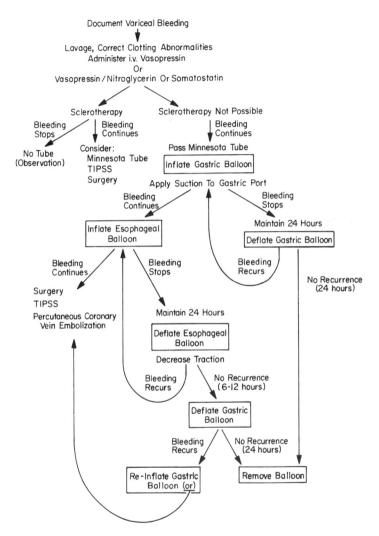

FIG. 2. Use of the Minnesota tube in a patient with variceal bleeding. TIPSS, transjugular intrahepatic portasystemic shunt.

particular risk if sclerotherapy has been performed prior to tube placement.

4. Cardiac arrhythmias.
5. Pulmonary edema.
6. Bronchopneumonia.

Minor

1. Unintentional deflation.
2. Inability to deflate because of cementing of the rubber-shod clamps.
3. Hiccoughs.
4. Agitation.

Efficacy

The Minnesota tube has been demonstrated to be better tolerated than the older Sengstaken-Blackmore tubes because of its softer rubber consistency. The Minnesota tube can be used safely in attaining initial hemostasis. The role of balloon tamponade is controversial. With the advent of improved sclerotherapy techniques, balloon tamponade has a limited role in the primary treatment of bleeding varices. Its greatest role may be in the tamponade of gastric varices as these are less accessible to sclerotherapy. In some series the Minnesota tube is also less efficacious in the treatment of gastric varices as compared to esophageal varices. The use of balloon tamponade may allow stabilization of a patient so that sclerotherapy or surgery becomes a treatment option. The overall outcome of hemorrhage control by either sclerotherapy or balloon tamponade is dependent on the underlying condition of the patient (12).

The effectiveness of balloon tamponade has ranged from 50% to 92% in the published series. The Minnesota tube has been shown to be equally effective as intravenous vasopressin in the cessation of esophageal variceal bleeding (13). Permanent cessation of bleeding occurs in 40% to 50% of patients treated with balloon tamponade. In one study efficacy depended on the degree of hypovolemia at presentation, those who required less than 1,500 cc of fluid resuscitation had a higher rate of successful tamponade (11). Long-term efficacy in terms of rebleeding is dependent in part on the patient's underlying liver disease. Only 25% patients with ascites, jaundice, and encephalopathy attain lasting hemostasis with balloon tamponade, whereas without these findings approximately 92% of patients will not rebleed (6).

REFERENCES

1. Mitchell K, Silk D, Williams R (1980): Prospective comparison of two Sengstaken tubes in the management of patients with variceal hemorrhage. *Gut* 21:570–573.
2. Edlich R, Lande A, Goodale R, *et al* (1968): Prevention of aspiration pneumonia by continuous esophageal aspiration during oesophagogastric tamponade and gastric cooling. *Surgery* 642:405–408.
3. Boyce HJ (1962): Modification of the Sengstaken-Blakemore balloon tube. *N Engl J Med* 267:195–196.
4. Westby D, Hayes P, Gimson A, *et al* (1989): Controlled clinical trial of injection sclerotherapy for active variceal bleeding. *Hepatology* 9:274–279.
5. Pitcher J (1967): Safety and effectiveness of the modified Sengstaken-Blakemore tube: a prospective study. *Gastroenterology* 61:291–298.
6. Novis B, Duys P, Barbezat G (1976): Fiberoptic endoscopy and the use of the Sengstaken tube in acute gastroesophageal hemorrhage from esophageal varices. *Gut* 17:258–263.
7. Conn H, Simpson J (1967): Excessive mortality associated with balloon tamponade of bleeding varices; a critical appraisal. *JAMA* 202:287–291.
8. Snow N, Almon M, Baillie J (1990): Minnesota tube placement using a guide wire. Letter. *Gastrointest Endosc* 36:420–421.
9. Kashiwagi H, Shikano S, Yamamoto O, *et al* (1991): Technique for positioning the Sengstaken-Blakemore tube as comfortably as possible. *Surg Gynecol Obstet* 172:63.
10. Fenig J, Richter R, Levowitz B (1976): Gastric ulceration caused by Sengstaken-Blakemore balloon tamponade. *NY State J Med* 76:404–407.
11. Panes J, Teres J, Bosch J, *et al* (1988): Efficacy of balloon tamponade in treatment of bleeding gastric and esophageal varices: results in 151 consecutive episodes. *Dig Dis Sci* 33:454–459.
12. Paquet K, Mercado M, Aichner W, *et al* (1990): Conservative and semi-invasive modalities for treating bleeding esophageal varices. *Hepatogastroenterology* 37:561–564.
13. Pinto-Correia J, Martins-Alves M, Alexandrino P, *et al* (1984): Controlled trial of vasopressin and balloon tamponade in acute hemorrhage from esophagogastric varices: a prospective controlled randomized trial. *Hepatology* 5:580–583.

4 / Esophageal Manometry

Roy C. Orlando

Esophageal manometry is a widely used procedure for the diagnosis and study of esophageal motor disorders (1). The reasons for its popularity are many; among them are the frequency with which patients have symptoms appropriate for study, the case and safety of performing the test, and the durability and low cost of maintaining the equipment. In recent times, the field of motility has moved from an art to a scientifically based area of investigative work with clinical application (2–4).

Indications

1. To evaluate patients with dysphagia and/or chest pain for esophageal motor disease.
2. To aid in the diagnosis of progressive systemic sclerosis (scleroderma) or intestinal pseudoobstruction by documenting esophageal motor dysfunction (1).
3. To evaluate the effectiveness of pneumatic dilatation or surgical myotomy in lowering the lower esophageal sphincter pressure (LESP) of patients with achalasia.
4. To evaluate esophageal motility and LESP prior to fundoplication (antireflux surgery) in patients with gastroesophageal reflux and to assess its effectiveness in raising LESP.
5. To localize the lower esophageal sphincter (LES) for positioning of pH probes, perfusion orifices, and biopsy ports.

Contraindications

1. Poor patient cooperation.
2. Patients with cardiac instability or other conditions in which vagal stimulation is poorly tolerated.

Preparation

1. Nothing by mouth for 6 to 8 hr before study.
2. Obtain written consent.

Equipment

1. A triple-lumen polyvinyl catheter assembly (Fig. 1) (internal diameter 1.1 mm) with 1-mm lateral sensing orifices spaced 5 cm apart (Arndorfer Medical Specialties Company, Greendale, Wisconsin). Alternative: solid-state manometry catheter system (Konigsberg Instruments, Pasadena, California) that contains four miniature pressure transducers, including one (the most distal) that senses pressure circumferentially over 360° (5).
2. Pneumohydraulic capillary infusion system (Arndorfer Medical Specialties Company, Greendale, Wisconsin)—perfusion rate 0.6 ml/min. Alternative: Harvard pump or other fluid delivery system with well-greased glass syringes to reduce compliance (2–4).
3. Multichannel recording system (Hewlett Packard Model No. 7758A, Hewlett Packard Company, Palo Alto, California) for use at paper speeds of 1 and 2.5 mm/sec. Alternative: similar equipment available from Beckman Instruments Inc.,

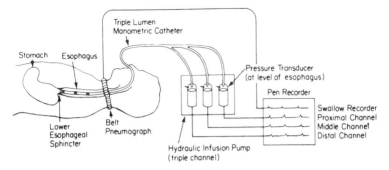

FIG. 1. Performance of esophageal manometry on supine subject using a standard triple-lumen perfused catheter assembly. *Note.* The pressure transducers (more specifically, the diaphragm within the head of the transducer) must be located at the level of the esophagus (midaxillary line) for optimum recording of absolute pressures.

Schiller Park, Illinois, and Honeywell Biomedical Instrumentation, Denver, Colorado.

4. Pressure transducers for each channel (Model No. 1280C, Hewlett Packard Company, Palo Alto, California). Alternative: similar equipment available from Beckman Instruments Inc., Schiller Park, Illinois, and Honeywell Biomedical Instrumentation, Denver, Colorado.

5. Swallowing sensor (bellows, sound or myoelectric type) (Beckman Instruments Inc., Schiller Park, Illinois; Hewlett Packard Company, Palo Alto, California).

6. Catheter-tipped syringe (10–50 cc) for wet swallows.

Procedure[1]

Calibration

1. Calibrate recording system according to manufacturer's directions.

2. Check the accuracy of the fluid-filled pressure transducer and recorder by attaching a sphygmomanometer to each pressure transducer (one at a time or by using an adapter to all three simultaneously) and noting the deflection of the recording needle as the sphygmomanometer is pumped up. *Note.* The needle will respond differently depending on the pressure range selected on the recorder. When testing the system on the 0 to 80 mm Hg scale, pump the sphygmomanometer to approximately 40 mm Hg. The needle should deflect an appropriate number of boxes to reflect this pressure. Repeat this sequence for each pressure range to be used.

3. Following calibration, check the pressure response rate of the system (a measure of its sensitivity to pressure changes within the esophagus) in the following way. Set the recorder on the highest pressure scale and start the fluid delivery pump running at normal speed (0.6 ml/min for Arndorfer pump) with the manometric catheters connected. When water completely fills a catheter and begins to flow from the distal orifice, completely occlude the orifice with your finger. Since the needle deflection produced is a measure of pressure and the paper speed allows a calculation of time, the

---

[1]For another detailed account see ref. 6 (Chapter 5. pp 41–51).

pressure response rate can be calculated in mm Hg/sec. Response rates ≥ 150 mm Hg/sec are acceptable for ensuring high-fidelity recordings from the lower and middle third (body) of the esophagus. *Note*. Response rates achievable by perfused catheter systems are inadequate for accurate pressure readings in the upper third (skeletal muscle) of the esophagus, which includes the upper esophageal sphincter (UES). For high-fidelity pressure readings from this area, the Konigsberg motility probe is recommended. The major advantages of perfused catheter systems over the motility probe are their flexibility (the number and location of recording orifices can be readily varied—ideal for research) and low replacement costs.

Clinical Study

After calibration, the clinical study is performed by passing the triple-lumen catheter via nose or mouth (nose preferable because of less gagging after passage) into the esophagus (see chapter by Reinhold and Nuzum) and advancing it until all channels record gastric pressure. Gastric pressure is indicated by regular low-amplitude waves whose amplitude can be increased by deep inspiration but is unaffected by swallowing (Fig. 2). The absolute gastric pressure usually ranges from 5 to 10 mm Hg when the pressure transducers are correctly located at the level of the esophagus.

Patient Placement

Place the patient in a supine position with arms at sides and attach the swallowing sensor to the neck.

Identify Lower Esophageal Sphincter

With the paper speed set at 1 mm/sec and the recorder on the lowest pressure scale (e.g., 0–80 mm Hg range on Hewlett Packard recorder):

1. Slowly withdraw the catheter assembly until a rise in baseline pressure is noted on the proximal channel. This pressure

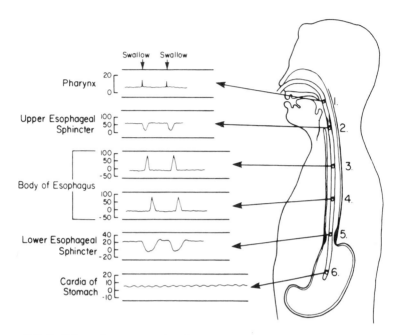

FIG. 2. Schematic representation of the intraluminal pressure events obtained at various points at rest and during swallows in a healthy subject. Pressure scales are in mm Hg.

rise should correspond to the LESP. This is verified by eliciting relaxation with swallows (Fig. 2).

2. Pull-through the LES at ½-cm intervals (station pull-through technique) until all three catheters have traversed it. The LES should appear at each orifice in sequence, approximately 5 cm apart. *Note.* The maximum pressure recorded within the LES may vary considerably for each channel (this reflects differences in spatial orientation of the channels and the asymmetry of the LES muscle). Some laboratories prefer to use a rapid pull-through technique for obtaining LES pressure (7), though current data do not support this method as being superior to the station pull-through technique. When each channel has passed through the LES, it enters the esophagus.

3. Location of the catheter within the esophagus is indicated by

a negative baseline pressure, reflecting intrathoracic pressure, and significant positive pressure waves on swallowing (Fig. 2).

Reposition Catheter Assembly

Reposition the catheter assembly with the distal channel recording from the zone of greatest LES pressure, then fix the assembly in place by taping to the nose. Have the subject swallow two to three times, then adjust the pressure range selector for each channel so that the highest pressures generated remain on scale. Record the proper pressure range for each channel on the manometric paper. Allow 5 min for subjects to adjust to the catheter assembly before formal testing.

Record LES and Esophageal Pressures

Administer a minimum of ten wet swallows (5 cc water given via syringe) at 1- to 2-min intervals. This recording provides information about LES pressure, LES relaxation, peristaltic complexes, and spontaneous contractions in the esophageal body.

After the last wet swallow, remove tape and reposition the catheter assembly with all three channels recording from the esophageal body. This is done by pulling it up 2 to 3 cm above the LES. Retape to the nose.

Perform another 5 to 10 wet swallows in this second position. This recording provides additional information about contractions in the body of the esophagus. In some patients, further sequential withdrawal of the catheter assembly at 1-cm increments, with swallows at each station, can aid in assessing the motor function of the entire esophageal body. This, however, is not generally necessary for diagnosing a motor disorder in most patients.

Upper Esophageal Sphincter

1. Remove tape and slowly withdraw the catheter assembly until the proximal channel encounters another high-pressure zone; this is UES. The UES can be verified by eliciting relaxation with swallows, similar to that seen with the LES.

2. Stop perfusion of the proximal channel. This helps to avoid minor aspiration and coughing. Continue the station pull-through until the middle channel records the UES. The proximal channel is now recording pharyngeal contractions and the distal channel is recording from the upper portion of the esophagus.
3. Switch the paper speed to 2.5 mm/sec. (This spreads the complexes, allowing coordination between UES relaxation and pharyngeal contraction to be more easily determined.)
4. With the catheter assembly fixed in this third position, perform 5 to 10 "dry" swallows.

Provocative Testing

For selected patients with unexplained chest pain and/or dysphagia, provocative testing may aid in the diagnosis of symptomatic esophageal motor disease. Such testing is appropriate (a) when routine esophageal manometric, radiologic, and endoscopic studies, and, for patients with chest pain, cardiac studies have failed to clarify the cause for symptoms; and (b) when there is evidence of impaired function despite adequate reassurance. Patients to be tested must also have no contraindication to the administration of a drug with cholinergic properties. Based on available efficacy and safety data (8,9), intravenous edrophonium chloride (Tensilon, Roche Laboratories, Nutley, New Jersey) is the drug of choice for provocative testing.

1. After routine manometry, reposition the catheter assembly as described earlier in this chapter.
2. Insert a No. 21 gauge scalp vein needle (E-Z 21 infusion set, Deseret Pharmaceutical Company, Inc., Sandy, Utah) into an accessible vein on the upper extremity. Flush tubing with sterile saline.
3. Check to see that atropine is on hand to reverse untoward effects from edrophonium administration.
4. Administer randomly either placebo (1 ml sterile saline fluid) or edrophonium (80 μg/kg; 10 mg maximal dose) as a rapid intravenous injection.
5. Perform ten wet swallows over a 5-min period and record patient symptoms on tracing.

6. Repeat step 4 using the alternate agent, placebo or edrophonium, as an intravenous bolus.
7. Repeat step 5 by performing ten wet swallows over 5 min and recording patient symptoms on tracing.
8. Interpretation. A positive test result occurs when injection of edrophonium, but not placebo, elicits the patient's chest pain *and* a manometric abnormality not observed on baseline testing.

Remove Catheter

Remove the catheter to conclude the study or leave it in place for pH probe testing (see chapter by Bozymski and Orlando), or Bernstein testing [see chapter by Sandler, "Bernstein (Acid Perfusion) Test"].

Postprocedure

Patient may resume normal activities.

Complications

None reported with routine manometry. For provocative testing with edrophonium, drug side effects reported include dizziness, nausea, and abdominal cramps.

Interpretation

Figure 2 shows a schematic representation of the motility pattern elicited by swallows in a healthy subject.

Esophageal Manometric Data

Esophageal manometric data obtained in "normal subjects" (25) at North Carolina School of Medicine, 14 female, 11 male, ages 21 to 36, mean age 26. No history of systemic disease, GI disorders, medication, heartburn, dysphagia, chest pain, or odynophagia.

Instruments Used

Perfused-catheter system (1.1 mm ID), three catheters with lateral sensing orifices 5 cm apart, perfusion rate 0.6 ml/min. External transducers (Hewlett Packard Company 1280C). Recorder/amplifier (Sanborn 7700 series), paper speed 1 mm/sec. Pneumohydraulic capillary infusion system (Arndorfer Medical Specialties Company, Greendale, Wisconsin). Belt pneumograph for swallows. Recording period 16 min with distal channel recording LES; middle and proximal channels 5 and 10 cm above LES in body, respectively.

Standard Data (Means ± SD)

Lower esophageal sphincter

1. LESP—mean 19.2 ± 6.9 mm Hg; range 9 to 32 mm Hg with peak = 11 to 40 mm Hg.
2. % LES relaxation (wet swallows)—mean 96 ± 10%; range of means 67% to 100%.

Esophageal body: primary peristalsis

1. Mean amplitude (wet swallows):
   a. Proximal channel—71 ± 26 mm Hg.
   b. Middle channel—65 ± 19 mm Hg.
2. Range of mean amplitudes (wet swallows):
   a. Proximal channel—35 to 120 mm Hg.
   b. Middle channel—27 to 100 mm Hg.
3. Mean duration (wet swallows):
   a. Proximal channel—4.8 ± 0.9 sec.
   b. Middle channel—4.8 ± 1.0 sec.
4. Range of mean duration (wet swallows):
   a. Proximal channel—3.3 to 6.2 sec.
   b. Middle channel—3.3 to 6.6 sec.
5. Propulsive versus nonpropulsive (simultaneous) contractions— 94.5% propulsive and 5.5% nonpropulsive with wet swallows.

Esophageal body: primary peristalsis

1. Mean amplitude (dry swallows):

    a. Proximal channel—45 ± 21 mm Hg.
    b. Middle channel—46 ± 13 mm Hg.
2. Range of mean amplitudes (dry swallows):
    a. Proximal channel—21 to 112 mm Hg.
    b. Middle channel—25 to 81 mm Hg.
3. Mean duration (dry swallows):
    a. Proximal channel—4.7 ± 0.9 sec.
    b. Middle channel—4.8 ± 0.8 sec.
4. Range of mean duration (dry swallows):
    a. Proximal channel—2.8 to 6.3 sec.
    b. Middle channel—3.4 to 6.3 sec.
5. Propulsive vs nonpropulsive (simultaneous)—84% propulsive and 16% nonpropulsive with dry swallows.

Esophageal body: tertiary contractions

1. Present in 22/25 or 88% of subjects.
2. Proximal channel—number of tertiary waves ranged 0 to 52 in 16-min recording.
3. Middle channel—number of tertiary waves ranged 0 to 64 in 16-min recording.
4. Tertiary contractions were "infrequent" in 18/25 or 72%— i.e., < 1 tertiary wave per minute.
5. Tertiary contractions were "frequent" in 7/25 or 28%—i.e., > 1 tertiary wave per minute.
    a. Range of frequency was 16 to 116 waves/16 min.
    b. Runs of 2 and 3 waves common; runs of 6 and 8 waves seen in two different subjects; no symptoms in any subject.
6. Mean amplitude:
    a. Proximal channel—12 ± 3 mm Hg.
    b. Middle channel—12 ± 3 mm Hg.
7. Mean duration:
    a. Proximal channel—3.1 ± 0.5 sec.
    b. Middle channel—2.9 ± 0.4 sec.

Note. Amplitude of tertiary contractions significantly lower than amplitude of primary peristaltic waves and duration of tertiary contractions significantly shorter than primary peristaltic waves.

Figures 3 to 5 illustrate schematically some characteristic mo-

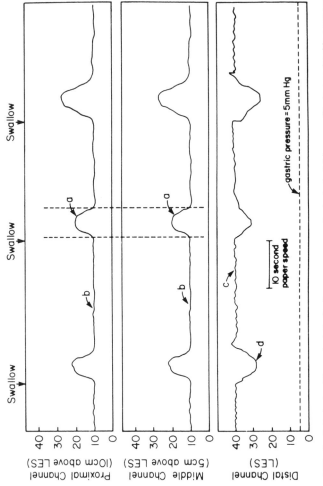

FIG. 3. Achalasia. Characteristic findings on manometry include (a) low-amplitude aperistaltic contractions with *all* swallows; (b) high resting pressure in the esophageal body; (c) high LES pressure; and (d) incomplete LES relaxation. For technical reasons, LES relaxation may appear complete on manometry in some subjects (1,11,12).

46

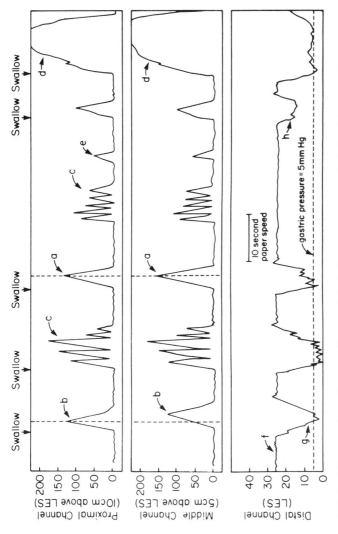

FIG. 4. Diffuse esophageal spasm. Characteristic findings on manometry include (a) increased frequency of aperistaltic contractions on swallowing; (b) some peristaltic contractions on swallowing; (c) repetitive contractions; (d) high-amplitude long-duration contractions; and (e) tertiary waves. The LES may have (f) normal pressure; high pressure (not shown); (g) complete relaxation on swallowing; or (h) incomplete relaxation on swallowing (1,11).

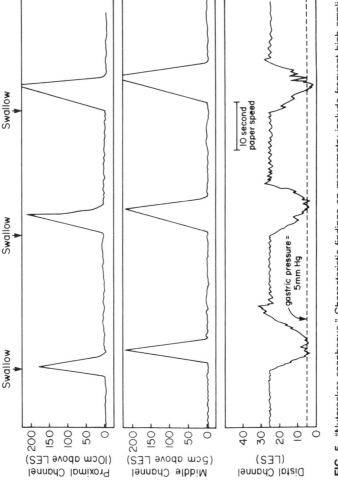

FIG. 5. "Nutcracker esophagus." Characteristic findings on manometry include frequent high-amplitude peristaltic contractions on swallowing (mean amplitude >120 mm Hg and/or peak amplitude of a single contraction >200 mm Hg). The duration of such contractions is usually prolonged, but this is not essential for the diagnosis. The LES is of normal pressure and relaxes completely on swallowing (1,11).

tor patterns in patients with symptomatic esophageal motor disease.

For provocative testing, see Provocative Testing section earlier in this chapter.

REFERENCES

1. Cohen S (1979): Motor disorders of the esophagus. *N Engl J Med* 301: 44–52.
2. Stef JJ, Dodds WJ, Hogan WJ, Linehan JH (1974): Esophageal manometry. Component analysis of systems used to record intraluminal pressure. *Proceedings of the Fourth International Symposium on Gastrointestinal Motility*, pp 337–346, Banff, Alberta, Canada.
3. Stef JJ, Dodds WJ, Hogan WJ, Linehan JH, Stewart ET (1974): Intraluminal esophageal manometry: an analysis of variables affecting recording fidelity of peristaltic pressures. *Gastroenterology* 67:221–230.
4. Arndorfer RC, Stef JJ, Dodds WJ, Linehan JH, Hogan WJ (1977): Improved infusion system for intraluminal esophageal manometry. *Gastroenterology* 73:23–37.
5. Castell JA, Dalton CB (1992): Esophageal manometry. In: *The Esophagus*, edited by DO Castell, pp 143–160. Little, Brown and Company, Boston.
6. Hurwitz AL, Duranceau A, Haddad JK (1979): Esophageal manometric technique; and the performance of the esophageal motility study. In: *Disorders of Esophageal Motility*, edited by LH Smith Jr, pp 27–51. WB Saunders Company, Philadelphia.
7. Dodds WJ, Hogan WJ, Stef JJ, Miller WN, Lydon AB, Arndorfer RC (1975): A rapid pull-through technique for measuring lower esophageal sphincter pressure. *Gastroenterology* 68:437–443.
8. Richter JE, Hackshaw BT, Wu WC, Castell DO (1985): Edrophonium: a useful provocative test for esophageal chest pain. *Ann Intern Med* 103: 14–21.
9. Benjamin SB, Richter JE, Cordova CM, Knuff TE, Castell DO (1983): Prospective manometric evaluation with pharmacologic provocation of patients with suspected esophageal motility dysfunction. *Gastroenterology* 84:893–901.
10. Benjamin SB, Gerhardt DC, Castell DO (1979): High amplitude, peristaltic esophageal contractions associated with chest pain and/or dysphagia. *Gastroenterology* 77:478–483.
11. Vantrappen G, Hellemans J (1982): Esophageal motor disorders. In: *Diseases of the Esophagus*, edited by S Cohen, RD Soloway, pp 161–179. Churchill Livingstone, New York.
12. Katz PO, Richter JE, Cowan R, Castell DO (1986): Apparent complete lower esophageal sphincter relaxation achalasia. *Gastroenterology* 90: 978–983.

5 / Ambulatory Intraesophageal pH Monitoring

Eugene M. Bozymski and Roy C. Orlando

Prolonged ambulatory intraesophageal pH monitoring is the single best test for detecting episodes of gastroesophageal (acid) reflux. Because the patient is able to carry out his or her daily routine, the test detects reflux episodes under more physiologic conditions. Acid reflux is not necessarily pathologic since asymptomatic healthy subjects have reflux (defined as esophageal pH falling to <4) periodically throughout the day, and most often after meals. However, esophageal symptoms (heartburn) and/or esophagitis (inflammation and necrosis of the esophageal epithelium) may occur when there is prolonged contact of acid with esophageal epithelium. For this reason, prolonged ambulatory intraesophageal pH monitoring can be used to assess the risk for esophageal symptoms or damage based on the frequency and duration of esophageal acidification, and calculation of total acid contact time. In addition, esophageal ambulatory pH monitoring can be used to correlate symptoms with esophageal acidification. Further information on this technique and its interpretation is available elsewhere (1).

Indications

1. To assess the probability of a reflux-related disorder in patients with heartburn (or other reflux-related symptoms) that fail medical therapy.
2. To establish the presence or absence of a correlation between esophageal acidification and functional chest pain.
3. To assess the probability of a reflux-related disorder in pa-

tients with oropharyngeal (hoarseness, laryngitis) or pulmonary disease (wheezing, asthma, aspiration pneumonia).
4. To establish a baseline of total acid contact time among patients scheduled for antireflux surgery.
5. To assess (in those with a preoperative baseline study) the technical success or failure of antireflux surgery in patients with continued or new chest complaints.
6. To assess in infants a possible role for gastroesophageal reflux with apneic episodes or failure to thrive.

Contraindications

See chapter by Reinhold and Nuzum.

Preparation

1. Obtain informed consent.
2. Do not allow patient to ingest solids or liquids for at least 4 hr prior to passage of pH electrode. This minimizes vomiting and prevents buffering of gastric contents.
3. Discontinue all antireflux medication for 24 hr prior to study or, in the case of omeprazole, for 7 days prior to study unless the study is being performed to assess failure of medical therapy to control symptoms.

Equipment

1. Flexible pH microelectrode and reference electrode.
2. Calibration buffers (pH 7.0 and pH 1.0).
3. Ambulatory battery-powered (9 V) pH meter with microprocessor recording device (e.g., Synectics Digitrapper, Irving, Texas).
4. pH software (e.g., Synectics, Irving, Texas).
5. Computer with serial port for attachment and printer.

Procedure

1. Calibrate the pH electrode. This is done by first zeroing the digitrapper utilizing the software program (see supplier's in-

struction manual). After attaching the electrodes (both pH and reference) to the digitrapper, place both recording ends into a standard buffer of pH 7.0 and record baseline values 3 min. The display on the digitrapper should read close to pH 7.0. After washing the electrodes, repeat the maneuver using a standard buffer at pH 1.0. The digitrapper display should read close to pH 1.0.

2. Pass the pH electrode via the nares into the stomach (as instructed for nasogastric tube placement—see chapter by Reinhold and Nuzum) to ensure that gastric contents are acidic (pH ≤4).

3. Withdraw the pH electrode from the stomach slowly until the recording device lies within the esophagus, 5 cm above the lower esophageal sphincter (LES). *Note.* The LES location is established either by reference to a prior manometric study in the patient or by passing the pH probe under fluoroscopic guidance until it is located 5 cm proximal to the diaphragm or the inferior border of the cardiac silhouette.

4. Fix the pH electrode in place by taping to the nares and cheek. Tape it to the lower part of the neck after looping it over the ear and running it toward the recorder.

5. Connect the reference electrode to the skin of the chest, e.g., the area over the manubrium sterni, where it is less likely to be disturbed by the patient's movements.

6. Shave hair from the area and swab with alcohol to ensure good skin contact with the electrode.

7. Connect the wires running from the pH electrode and reference electrodes to the recording device, which is strapped around the waist or worn on a belt.

Patient Instructions

8. Diary. Instruct the patient on the proper method of keeping a diary for the study. This should include notations as to time and duration that the patient is:
   a. Upright—awake or asleep.
   b. Recumbent—awake or asleep.
   c. Eating (and types of foods consumed—see diet notation below).

   d. Smoking.

   e. Experiencing belching, hiccupping, vomiting, and coughing.

   f. Experiencing spontaneous chest symptoms.

9. Activities. Instruct the patient to resume his or her usual activities and to avoid getting the recording device wet.

10. Diet. In some centers the patient is instructed to avoid eating or drinking acidic foods (e.g., fruit juices, carbonated beverages, fruit, tomatoes or tomato-based foods, sauerkraut). Other centers prefer that the patient eat his or her normal diet since the diary will identify maladaptive eating habits. The patient should be instructed to drink only water between meals.

11. Smoking is permitted.

12. After recording for 16 to 24 hr, remove the pH and reference electrodes and download the recorder into the computer according to the software manufacturer's instructions.

13. After returning the diary, the patient can resume normal activities and restart discontinued medications.

Interpretation

1. Baseline data. The computerized record will generally provide the following:

   a. Frequency and duration of all reflux episodes (as defined by esophageal pH <4) over the monitored time period.

   b. Frequency and duration of reflux episodes in the upright or supine (recumbent) positions.

   c. Total acid contact time (frequency × duration summed for all reflux events).

   d. Frequency of reflux events lasting longer than 5 min.

2. Discrimination between physiologic and pathologic reflux. The software can also be used to assess the above parameters for a given time period, or assess the total record after deletion of a time period (for example, during the postprandial period where there are multiple episodes of reflux even in asymptomatic individuals). The results can then be interpreted to show physiologic reflux (i.e., a reflux pattern that falls within the range in normal healthy volunteers) or patho-

logic reflux (i.e., a reflux pattern that falls outside this physiologic range). Below are some values (2) commonly used to distinguish physiologic from pathologic reflux:

Parameter	Normal Range
Total no. reflux episodes	
Upright	<2.3/hr
Supine	<0.4/hr
Mean duration of episodes	
Upright	<1.6 min
Supine	<2.1 min
Number of episodes>5 min	
Upright	<2/24 hr
Supine	<1/24 hr
Duration—longest episode	
Upright	<11.5 min
Supine	<8.5 min
Overall	<11.5 min
Total time pH <4	
Upright	<10.5%
Supine	<6%

Note. When used together, total time pH <4 in upright position of 10.5% and total time pH <4 in supine position of 6% have a sensitivity of 93% and specificity of 93% in distinguishing between those with physiologic reflux and those with pathologic reflux. Although more elaborate scoring systems are sometimes used (1) to distinguish physiologic from pathologic reflux, these systems have not been uniformly effective in providing better discrimination.

3. Correlation of symptoms with reflux. By matching the computerized printout with the patient's diary, a correlation between esophageal acidification and spontaneous symptoms is also provided. A positive correlation exists when all spontaneous chest symptoms are associated with esophageal acidification (symptoms occur during esophageal acidification or within 1–2 min after an episode of acidification) and no symptoms occur in the absence of similar degrees of esophageal acidification. However, this is rarely achieved because

of the frequency of esophageal acidification in the absence of symptoms. The occurrence of symptoms during esophageal acidification, even when many similar episodes of esophageal acidification are asymptomatic, is often accepted as supporting a *possible* relationship.

REFERENCES

1. Richter JE (1991): *Ambulatory Esophageal pH Monitoring. Practical Approach and Clinical Applications.* Igaku-Shoin, New York.
2. Schindlbeck NE, Heinrich C, Konig A, Dendorfer A, Pace F, Muller-Lissner SA (1987): Optimal thresholds, sensitivity, and specificity of long-term pH metry for the detection of gastroesophageal reflux disease. *Gastroenterology* 93:85.

Recommended Reading

1. Mattox HE, Richter JE (1990): Prolonged ambulatory esophageal pH monitoring in the evaluation of gastroesophageal reflux disease. *Am J Med* 89:345–356.
2. Lieberman D (1988): 24-Hour esophageal pH monitoring before and after medical therapy for reflux esophagitis. *Dig Dis Sci* 33:166–171.
3. Rosen SN, Pope CN (1989): Extended esophageal pH monitoring: an analysis of the literature and assessment of its role in the diagnosis and management of gastroesophageal reflux. *J Clin Gastroenterol* 11:260.
4. McLauchlan G, Rawling JM, Lucal ML, et al (1987): Electrodes for 24 hr pH monitoring: a comparative study. *Gut* 28:935.

6 / Bernstein (Acid Perfusion) Test

Robert S. Sandler

The Bernstein test is a clinical procedure to identify esophageal acid sensitivity. The test was originally devised to distinguish between angina pectoris and esophageal pain in the patient with atypical chest pain (1). It currently finds its widest use in the evaluation of chest pain patients. Although the specificity is believed to be high (2), the sensitivity in patients with atypical chest pain is relatively low, ranging from 7% to 27% (3). Thus, while most patients with acid-related chest pain will not be diagnosed by the Bernstein test, a positive result strongly supports esophageal acid sensitivity (4). The value of the Bernstein and other provocative tests in elucidating the cause of atypical chest pain has been questioned (5).

The mechanism for pain production is uncertain but may be due to direct stimulation of exposed esophageal sensory receptors (6). Studies in patients with esophagitis have suggested that pH is not the sole factor responsible for heartburn (7). On the other hand, among patients with esophageal acid sensitivity there was a positive correlation between the time elapsed before pain perception and the pH of the solution infused (8). All patients experienced pain with pH <1.5 and 80% had pain with pH 2.0 solution.

The procedure appears to be quite safe. Acid perfusion does not produce gross esophagoscopic abnormalities. The test does not produce angina or esophageal bleeding. In patients with coronary artery disease, a positive Bernstein test may produce ST segment depression on EKG consistent with myocardial ischemia (9).

Indication

To determine if the patient's symptoms are due to esophageal acid sensitivity. The test evaluates symptoms alone and does not indicate the presence of esophagitis or acid reflux.

Contraindication

Active or recent bleeding from a peptic source.

Preparation of Patient

The patient should be fasting.

Equipment

1. Nasogastric (NG) tube (14–16 French). If the patient has undergone esophageal manometry, the manometry catheter may be used.
2. Three-way stopcock.
3. Reservoirs of normal saline solution and 0.1 N HCl.
4. Lubricant.

Procedure

1. Place the patient in an upright position (alternatively the procedure can be done with the patient recumbent).
2. Pass the lubricated NG tube (see chapter by Reinhold and Nuzum) so that the perfusing tip is 30 to 35 cm from the nares. If a manometry catheter is used, the perfusing orifice should be 5 cm above the manometrically identified lower esophageal sphincter.
3. Connect the NG tube to the reservoirs of 0.1 N HCl and normal saline solution via the three-way stopcock. Place the reservoirs behind the patient so that the flow can be switched without the patient's knowledge (Fig. 1).
4. Instruct the patient to indicate whether the drip produces typical symptoms or some new complaint.

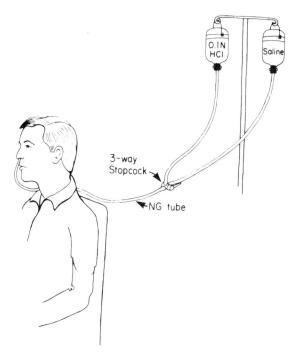

FIG. 1. Bernstein test. Solutions of 0.1 NHCl and saline solution are placed behind the patient. The flow can be switched by turning the three-way stopcock without the patient's knowledge.

5. Drip normal saline solution at 100 to 120 drops (6–7.5 ml) per minute for 5 min.
6. After 5 min, switch the flow to 0.1 N HCl using the three-way stopcock.
7. Allow the acid to flow until symptoms appear or until 30 min has elapsed. Disregard transient or momentary symptoms. Symptoms in a positive test are persistent and usually progressive in severity as long as administration of acid continues.
8. If symptoms appear, switch back to normal saline solution. The symptoms may decrease in 3 or 4 min. If the symptoms disappear with saline infusion, switch the flow back to 0.1 N HCl. The symptoms will reappear if they are due to esophageal sensitivity.

9. Record whether acid perfusion reproduces the patient's typical symptoms, results in heartburn, or produces a new sensation. All of these types of pain indicate a positive Bernstein test but have different implications. Confusion might result if the test is simply reported as positive without a description of the symptoms.

Interpretation

While the study is simple to perform, it may be difficult to interpret because it relies on the subjective responses of the patient. The test is positive if the patient reports discomfort during acid perfusion. Saline infusion may relieve the acid-induced symptoms but should not be required as a criterion for a positive test (10). If acid perfusion reproduces the patient's chest pain, then the test provides evidence for the esophageal origin of the complaints. If the patient complains of burning discomfort (heartburn) that is different from the patient's typical pain, the study indicates that the esophagus is sensitive to acid but does not help to evaluate the patient's symptoms of chest pain. If the patient complains of a new pain, the test is inconclusive.

REFERENCES

1. Bernstein LM, Baker LA (1958): A clinical test for esophagitis. *Gastroenterology* 34:760–781.
2. Richter JE, Bradley LA, Castell DO (1989): Esophageal chest pain: current controversies in pathogenesis, diagnosis and therapy. *Ann Intern Med* 110:66–78.
3. Katz DO, Dalton CB, Richter JE, Wu WC, Castell DO (1987): Esophageal testing in patients with noncardiac chest pain or dysphagia: results of three years' experience with 1161 patients. *Ann Intern Med* 106:593–597.
4. Richter JE, Hewson EG, Sinclair JW, Dalton CB (1991): Acid perfusion test and 24-hour esophageal pH monitoring with symptom index: comparison of tests for esophageal acid sensitivity. *Dig Dis Sci* 36:565–571.
5. Cohen S (1989): Noncardiac chest pain: the crumbling of the sphinx. *Dig Dis Sci* 34:1649–1650.
6. Dodds WJ, Hogan WJ, Miller WM (1976): Food sensitivity in reflux esophagitis. *Gastroenterology* 75:240–243.

7. Price SF, Smithson KW, Castell DO (1978): Food sensitivity in reflux esophagitis. *Gastroenterology* 75:240–243.
8. Smith JL, Opekun AR, Larkai E, Graham DY (1989): Sensitivity of the esophageal mucosa to pH in gastroesophageal reflux disease. *Gastroenterology* 96:683–689.
9. Mellow MH, Walt L, Haye O, et al (1981): Cardiovascular response to esophageal acid perfusion in coronary artery disease. *Gastroenterology* 80:1230.
10. Winnan GR, Meyer CT, McCallum RW (1982): Interpretation of the Bernstein test: a reappraisal of criteria. *Ann Intern Med* 96:320–322.

7 / Gastric Secretory Testing

Kenneth B. Klein

Gastric secretory testing assesses the basal and maximal capacity of the stomach to produce acid. Because of a number of important diagnostic and therapeutic advances in recent years, gastric secretory testing now has rather limited clinical usefulness.

As a screening test for the stomach's acid-producing capacity, some endoscopists measure the pH of a sample of gastric fluid obtained during upper gastrointestinal endoscopy. Although in general the lower the fasting pH, the greater the peak acid output, the relationship is rather variable and no studies have defined a fasting pH level that would reliably correspond to a hypersecretory state. On the other hand, the finding of a fasting pH of >5 in men and >7 in women [at least when the sample is obtained via nasogastric (NG) intubation after emptying the fasted stomach of residual fluid] appears to be a sensitive test of hypochlorhydria (1).

Indications

Helpful in Some Circumstances

1. In recurrent peptic ulcer disease, especially after ulcer surgery:
   a. To rule out hypersecretory states (e.g., Zollinger-Ellison syndrome, retained antrum).
   b. To test for completeness of vagotomy.
2. To determine the optimal dosage of acid-lowering drugs in Zollinger-Ellison syndrome.
3. To evaluate the patient with hypergastrinemia:

   a. Is it "pathological" (e.g., Zollinger-Ellison syndrome,
      G-cell hyperplasia)?
   b. Is it a physiological response to hypochlorhydria (e.g.,
      atrophic gastritis)?

Rarely Helpful

1. To establish the diagnosis of Zollinger-Ellison syndrome.
   Serum gastrin levels and gastrin response to secretin infusion
   have greater sensitivity and specificity than measurement of
   gastric acid secretion, even with determination of the basal
   acid output/maximal acid output (BAO/MAO) ratio (2,3).
2. To diagnose pernicious anemia. Serum B_{12} levels and the
   Schilling test are more specific; most cases of achlorhydria
   are not associated with pernicious anemia.
3. To predict the likelihood of ulcer recurrence after surgery.
   Measurement of either preoperative or postoperative acid secretion is in general not useful (4).

Virtually Never Helpful

1. For the evaluation of dyspepsia.
2. In the routine evaluation of patients with peptic ulcer disease.
3. To help determine the optimal type of ulcer surgery.
4. To distinguish benign from malignant gastric ulcers. Only
   20% of gastric cancers occur in the setting of achlorhydria
   (5). Furthermore, benign ulcers occasionally occur in stom-
   achs that produce little or no acid.

Contraindications

1. Gastric outlet obstruction.
2. Recent upper gastrointestinal bleeding.
3. Potential obstruction to free passage of an NG tube, such
   as prior nasopharyngeal surgery, Zenker's diverticulum, or
   high-grade esophageal stricture.
4. Upper respiratory infection or allergic rhinitis.

Preparation

1. Discontinue all medications that might affect gastric secretion at least 24 hr prior to testing. These include H_2 blockers, antihistamines, cholinergics, anticholinergics, tranquilizers, antidepressants, and carbonic anhydrase inhibitors. If the patient is experiencing peptic ulcer pain, antacids may be used for symptomatic relief during this period.
2. Give nothing by mouth after midnight.
3. Explain the nature of the procedure to the patient.

Equipment

1. A 14 to 18 French NG tube. A double- lumen (vented) tube is preferred.
2. Supplies for passing the tube (see chapter by Reinhold and Nuzum).
3. A 50- or 60-ml "catheter-tip" syringe.
4. Pentagastrin, 6 μg/kg, for parenteral injection.
5. Intermittent suction pump (desirable, but not essential).
6. Eight 120-cc fluid collection containers.
7. Acid titrating equipment, including a pH meter, graduated burette, small beakers, and 0.1 N NaOH.

Procedure

1. Introduce the NG tube into the nose and advance it until the tip lies in the stomach (see chapter by Reinhold and Nuzum).
2. Aspirate stomach contents. If food particles or more than a few hundred milliliters of fluid are present, the test should not be done, and the reason for this finding determined (e.g., the patient ate breakfast, gastric outlet obstruction, motility disorder).
3. Position the tip of the tube in the most dependent portion of the stomach. This may be determined by fluoroscopy or equally well by the "water-recovery test" (6,7). In this test, 20 to 50 ml of water is introduced into the stomach via the NG tube or by asking the patient to swallow it. Then, as much of the water as possible is aspirated through the tube

using the catheter-tip syringe. Placement is adequate if recovery is greater than 90%.

4. Collect gastric juice either by machine suction (preferably intermittent) or by frequent manual aspiration. Ensure tube patency by injecting small quantities of air every 5 min or so. Note the presence of blood or bile, either of which may result in erroneously low acid values.

5. For routine gastric analysis, it is not necessary to prevent the swallowing of sputum (e.g., by use of a dental sucker) or to use a marker to correct for gastric fluid loss through the pylorus. The patient may sit comfortably in a chair; precise positioning is not important (6).

6. *BAO collection.* Collect gastric secretions for the first hour in four 15-min samples.

7. *Pentagastrin injection.* After the first hour, inject pentagastrin, 6 μg/kg subcutaneously, which will maximally stimulate acid production (8). Warn the patient of these possible side effects: flushing, nausea, abdominal pain, dizziness, palpitations, and faintness (usually they are mild and transient).

8. *Peak acid output (PAO) collection.* During the postinjection hour, again collect gastric secretions in four 15-min samples.

9. Calculate BAO and PAO (see below).

Postprocedure

1. Repeat the water-recovery test to document that final tube placement was appropriate.
2. Aspirate any remaining gastric fluid.
3. Remove the NG tube.
4. Resume medications.

Interpretation: Measurement of Acid Content and Calculation of BAO and PAO

1. Measure and record the volume of each of the eight 15-min collections. (*Note.* Figure 1 is an example of a worksheet that we find useful in the recording and calculation of gastric secretory testing data.)

Patient Name: _____

Weight: _____ kg

Indication: _____

Patient #: _____

Date: _____ _____ _____
        M   D   Y

I. FIRST HOUR - BAO

Sample No	Scheduled Time (mins)	Actual Clock Time (0-2400) Start	Actual Clock Time (0-2400) End	Appearance	(a) Vol (mls)	(b) pH	(c) ml 0.1 N NaOH to pH 7.0 (5 ml aliquot)	(d) meq H⁺/ml Sample (c ÷ 50)	(e) meq H⁺/Total Sample (a x d)
1	0 - 15								
2	15 - 30								
3	30 - 45								
4	45 - 60								

BAO = Σ e = _____ meq H⁺/hr

II. SECOND HOUR - PAO and MAO

Pentagastin injection (6 µg/kg): _____ µg (_____ ml)

Time of injection: _____ (0-2400)

Sample No	Scheduled Time (mins)	Actual Clock Time (0-2400) Start	Actual Clock Time (0-2400) End	Appearance	(a) Vol (mls)	(b) pH	(c) ml 0.1 N NaOH to pH 7.0 (5 ml aliquot)	(d) meq H⁺/ml Sample (c ÷ 50)	(e) meq H⁺/Total Sample (a x d)
5	0 - 15								
6	15 - 30								
7	30 - 45								
8	45 - 60								

PAO = Two highest adjacent (e) column values x 2 = _____ meq H⁺/hr

MAO = Σ e = _____ meq H⁺/hr

Signature _____

FIG. 1. Gastric secretory testing worksheet.

TABLE 1. Gastric Secretory Testing: Typical Values

	BAO (mmol H$^+$/hr)		MAO (mmol H$^+$/hr)		PAO (mmol H$^+$/hr)	
	Average	Range	Average	Range	Average	Range
Normal subjects						
Males	2.5	0–10	25	7–50	35	10–60
Females	1.5	0–6	15	5–30	25	8–40
Duodenal ulcer						
Males	5.0	0.1–15	40	15–60	45	15–70
Females	3.0	0.1–15	30	10–45	35	15–55
Gastric ulcer						
Males	1.5	0–8	20	5–40		
Females	1.0	0–5	12	3–25		
Zollinger-Ellison syndrome, both sexes	40	10–90	65	30–120		

2. If particulate matter is present, centrifuge the sample.
3. An aliquot (e.g., 5 ml) from each of the eight collections is then titrated with 0.1 N NaOH to pH 7.0.
4. Calculate the acid content of each 15-min collection as follows:
   a. (ml NaOH needed for titration to pH 7.0) × 0.1 = mmol H$^+$ in aliquot
   b. mmol H$^+$ in 15-min collection
   $$= \frac{\text{volume of collection}}{\text{volume of aliquot}} \times \text{mmol H}^+ \text{ in aliquot}$$
5. BAO, expressed as mmol H$^+$/hr, is the sum of the acid content of the four 15-min collections made during the first hour.
6. PAO, expressed as mmol H$^+$/hr, is determined by adding the acid content of the two adjacent 15-min postpentagastrin collections with the highest values, then multiplying by 2. PAO represents the greatest acid output of which the parietal cell mass is capable. It is also the most reproducible of the various measures of acid stimulation (8).
7. MAO, expressed mmol H$^+$/hr, has been defined in various ways but is generally taken to represent the sum of the acid content of the four 15-min collections following pentagastrin administration.
8. See Table 1 for representative values.

REFERENCES

1. Feldman M, Barnett C (1991): Fasting gastric pH and its relationship to true hypochlorhydria in humans. *Dig Dis Sci* 36:866–869.
2. Malagelada JR, Davis CS, O'Fallon WM, Go VLW (1982): Laboratory diagnosis of gastrinoma: I. a prospective evaluation of gastric analysis and fasting serum gastrin levels. *Mayo Clin Proc* 57:211–218.
3. Malagelada JR, Glanzman SC, Go VLW (1982): Laboratory diagnosis of gastrinoma: II. a prospective study of gastrin challenge tests. *Mayo Clin Proc* 57:219–226.
4. Johnston D, Pickford IR, Walker BE, Goligher JC (1975): Highly selective vagotomy for duodenal ulcer: do hypersecretors need antrectomy? *Br Med J* 1:716–718.
5. Baron JH (1979): Gastric ulcer and carcinoma. In: *Clinical Tests of Gastric Secretion: History, Methodology, and Interpretation*, pp 86–97. Oxford University Press, New York.
6. Hassan MA, Hobsley M (1970): Positioning of subject and of nasogastric tube during a gastric secretory study. *Br Med J* 1:458–460.
7. Findlay JM, Prescott RJ, Sircus W (1972): Comparative evaluation of water recovery test and fluoroscopic screening in positioning a nasogastric tube during gastric secretory studies. *Br Med J* 4:458–461.
8. Baron JH (1979): Maximal stimuli. In: *Clinical Tests of Gastric Secretion: History, Methodology, and Interpretation*, pp 25–35. Oxford University Press, New York.

8 / Secretin Test

Roy C. Orlando

The pancreas, by virtue of its location, has been a difficult organ to study. Nonetheless, for over 35 years, the availability of the secretin test has helped diagnose chronic pancreatitis and pancreatic cancer in many patients (1–3). Since the advent of ultrasonography, computerized axial tomography, arteriography, and endoscopic retrograde cholangiopancreatography, reliance on the secretin test to diagnose these conditions has appropriately diminished. Yet the test remains important as a method for obtaining pancreatic cytologic specimens and documenting abnormalities in pancreatic exocrine function.

Indications

For evaluating patients with abdominal pain, weight loss, or steatorrhea in whom the diagnosis of chronic pancreatitis or pancreatic cancer is suspected.

Contraindications

1. Acute pancreatitis.
2. Uncooperative patient.
3. Allergy to secretin.

Preparation

1. Give nothing by mouth after midnight.
2. Obtain informed, written consent.

Equipment

1. Dreiling tube (Davol Rubber Company): a double-lumen tube with one set of aspiration ports positioned to retrieve gastric contents and the other for duodenal contents.
2. Secretin-Kabi (Greenwich, Connecticut): same as secretin-GIH. Replaces secretin-Boots, which is a less-pure formulation with greater potential for allergic reactions.
3. Collection bottles.
4. Basin with ice.
5. Two 50-cc catheter-tipped syringes for aspirating gastric and duodenal juice and one 10-cc syringe for administering secretin.
6. pH paper.
7. No. 21 gauge scalp vein needle and tubing.
8. Suction units: wall or portable.
9. Fluoroscopy unit.

Procedure

1. The Dreiling tube is passed by mouth into the stomach and then guided with the aid of fluoroscopy through the duodenum to the ligament of Treitz.
2. With the patient supine and the tube in proper position (Fig. 1), aspirate juice from the duodenal and gastric channels using different 50-cc syringes. The duodenal juice should be alkaline and usually bile stained, whereas the gastric juice should be acidic (check with pH paper).
3. After verifying that the tube is properly positioned, tape it to the nose and aspirate gastric contents until there is no return.
4. Collection of baseline sample:
   a. Connect both gastric and duodenal channels to a suction unit for continuous low suctioning at 25 to 40 mm Hg for 10 to 20 min.
   b. Discard gastric juice.
   c. The duodenal juice collected is the basal sample.
   d. Measure its total volume; then handle the sample as described in item 6.f (below).

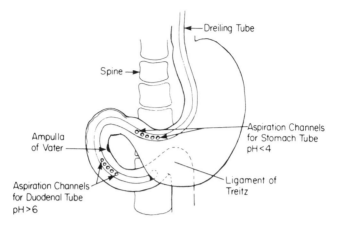

FIG. 1. Schematic representation of a Dreiling tube properly positioned for performance of the secretin test. *Note.* All gastric aspiration ports are within the stomach, and all duodenal ports are distal to the pylorus such that they only aspirate duodenal contents.

    c. Reinstitute suctioning of both gastric and duodenal secretions.

5. Administer secretin-Kabi 0.1 CU intravenously (i.v.) to test for allergy. If there is no reaction after 1 min, then administer the full dose of 1 CU/kg i.v. over 1 min.

6. Collection of stimulated samples:

    a. Immediately begin to collect the first of four consecutive 20-min samples (labeled in order) by continuous suctioning of duodenal contents.

    b. Measure the total volume for each sample before placing part of the sample into a collection tube for bicarbonate (HCO_3^-) determination. *Note.* Tubes should be kept on ice until ready for processing.

    c. Repeat for each sample.

    d. Pool the remaining fluid from each sample and place it in a beaker on ice for cytologic study.

    e. After collecting all four samples, remove the Dreiling tube by slow withdrawal.

    f. *Immediately* take the samples for cytology and HCO_3^- determination to their respective laboratories for processing. *Note.* The chemistry request slip *must* indicate that HCO_3^- determinations need to be carried out accurately; i.e., dilutions need to be made to obtain the final concentration of HCO_3^-. If this is not done, HCO_3^- will be reported as >40 mEq/liter, a level that has no diagnostic value.

TABLE 1. Secretin Test Results for Diagnosing Chronic Pancreatitis and Pancreatic Cancer

	Diagnosis	
	Chronic Pancreatitis	Pancreatic Cancer
Cytology	Negative	Positive (60% of cases)
HCO_3^-	<90 mEq/liter in all samples	≥90 mEq/liter in one or more samples
Total volume[a]	≥2 ml/kg	<2 ml/kg

[a]Sum of all sample volumes after secretin divided by weight in kilograms.

Postprocedure

The patient may resume normal activities.

Interpretation

Although earlier versions of the secretin test included amylase assays, these have been omitted here because of their limited value in diagnosing chronic pancreatitis and pancreatic cancer.

Pitfalls Affecting Results

1. Inadequate aspiration of gastric contents can lead to acidification of the duodenal juice, producing falsely low HCO_3^-.
2. Inadequate collection of duodenal contents can lead to falsely low total volume.
3. Poor tube position can cause errors in HCO_3^- and/or volume.
4. Patients with prior vagotomy, with inflammatory bowel disease, or currently on anticholinergic therapy may have low values in the absence of pancreatic pathology.

5. Except for a *positive* cytology result, which is conclusive for cancer, the data obtained (i.e., volume and HCO_3^-) should be viewed as objective evidence in support of chronic pancreatitis or pancreatic cancer. However, since the patterns shown may overlap in approximately 5% of cases, these findings are not pathognomonic for these disorders.

Complications

Allergic reactions (secretin-Boots)—none reported with secretin-Kabi.

REFERENCES

1. Dreiling DA (1975): Pancreatic secretory testing. *Gut* 16:653–657.
2. Banks PA (1979): Diagnosis of chronic pancreatitis. In: *Pancreatitis*, edited by HM Spiro, pp 202–204. Plenum Medical Book Company, New York.
3. Brooks FP (1980): Chronic and chronic relapsing pancreatitis. In: *Diseases of the Exocrine Pancreas*, edited by LH Smith Jr, pp 51–54. WB Saunders Company, Philadelphia.

9 / Rectal Manometry and Biofeedback Therapy

Robert S. Sandler

Rectal manometry is a technique used to record pressures from the rectum and the anal sphincters. The procedure is typically used to evaluate patients with constipation and fecal incontinence. The equipment may also be used to provide biofeedback training that may prove useful in patients with constipation due to spastic pelvic floor and in those with fecal incontinence from many causes.

Indications

1. To exclude Hirschsprung's disease in patients with long-standing constipation.
2. Evaluation and biofeedback training for fecal incontinence.
3. Evaluation and biofeedback training in adults with constipation from spastic pelvic floor (pelvic floor dyssynergia) and encopretic children with abnormal defecation dynamics.
4. To evaluate patients who have undergone ileoanal pull-through surgery prior to restoration of bowel continuity.

Contraindications

None.

Preparation

Generally no preparation is necessary. If a large amount of hard stool is present or anticipated, administer a rectal enema.

Equipment

Nonperfused Rectal Manometry Apparatus (Fig. 1)

The system consists of a doughnut-shaped balloon that records from the internal sphincter and a pear-shaped balloon that measures pressures from the subcutaneous bundle of the external sphincter. The balloon apparatus is commercially available (Sandhill Scientific, Littleton, Colorado; E.J. McGowan & Associates, Elmhurst, Illinois). Both disposable and reusable devices can be purchased.

Perfused Catheter System

Rectal manometry can also be performed using a multilumen polyvinyl catheter assembly with 1-mm lateral sensing orifices that are perfused with water by means of a low-compliance pneumohydraulic capillary infusion system. The catheters are similar to those used for esophageal manometry (see chapter by Orlando, "Esophageal Manometry") but are modified to include a rectal distending balloon at the distal tip (Arndorfer Medical Specialties, Inc., Greendale, Wisconsin, or Mui Scientific, Mississauga, Ontario, Canada).

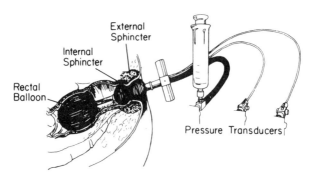

FIG. 1. The apparatus used for rectal manometry is shown in position. Each balloon is linked to a separate pressure transducer. Distension of the rectal balloon with air elicits the rectosphincteric response.

Solid-State Systems and Electromyographic Plugs

Solid-state microtransducer systems are available for rectal manometry. The transducers are built into the catheter, thereby eliminating the need for perfusion pumps and separate transducers. These are often linked to computers for data storage and output. Electromyographic (EMG) plugs are devices that are particularly valuable for biofeedback. They consist of plastic plugs with silver electrodes that sample activity from the anal sphincter muscles (Synectics, Irving, Texas). An advantage of the plugs is that they do not sense contraction of the buttocks and therefore provide more specific information about activity within the anus. Moreover, they can provide simple feedback to the patient, either audibly or visually. Portable devices that patients can use at home to practice anal sphincter contractions are available.

Recorder

A multichannel pen recorder or computer system is necessary to record the manometric tracing. There must be at least three channels, each connected to a pressure transducer.

Additional Equipment

The additional equipment needed depends on the type of apparatus used. In general, the following will be necessary.

1. Exam gloves.
2. Lubricant.
3. Gauze pads, 4 × 4 in.
4. Towels and gowns.
5. Sterile disposable needle.

Procedure

The following are general suggestions. Minor modifications may be necessary depending on the specific equipment used. Before performing this procedure, one should obtain hands-on supervised training from someone experienced in manometry. A videotape entitled "Biofeedback Treatment of Fecal Incontinence" can be obtained from National Audiovisual Center (8700 Edgeworth Drive, Capitol Heights, Maryland 20743-4701), and workshops are periodically available.

Nonperfused System

1. Prior to the procedure, make sure that the system is airtight by inflating the sphincter balloons under water with 10 cc of air and the rectal balloon with 50 cc of air for 30 sec.
2. Attach the three polyethylene catheters to the pressure transducers.
3. Lubricate the balloons.
4. The patient should lie on the left side with knees bent. Carefully inspect the perineum and perianal area. Retract the buttocks to determine if the anal sphincter gapes. Check pinprick sensation bilaterally using the disposable needle and note the presence or absence of an anal wink. Ask the patient to perform the Valsalva maneuver to assess perineal descent. Do a careful rectal examination. Ask the patient to contract the anus, noting the tone and response of the pelvic muscles.
5. Insert the apparatus following distension of the anus with a gloved finger.
6. Advance the rectal balloon about 7 to 8 cm.
7. Advance the cylinder with its sensing balloons until the external balloon can barely be seen.
8. Inflate the internal balloon with 8 cc of air. This will usually pull the apparatus into the rectum and will be felt as a tug on the cylinder. If inflation of the internal balloon results in movement of the apparatus out of the anus, deflate the balloon and insert the cylinder a little farther before reinflating.
9. Inflate the external balloon with 8 cc of air so that it is partially visible protruding from the anus.
10. Inflate the rectal balloon with 30 cc of air two or three times to seat the apparatus and to assess patency of the system.
11. If necessary, adjust the baseline of the recorder so that the tracings are centered. Calibration of resting pressure is not crucial. The pressures recorded by balloons are not an accurate reflection of sphincter pressures because of distortion of the anatomy by the balloons. The recorder should be cali-

brated to 10 mm Hg/cm and paper speed should be set at 1 mm/sec.

12. *Internal sphincter relaxation.* Inflate the rectal balloon with 30 to 50 cc of air to evaluate the response of the internal sphincter to rectal distension. The internal sphincter should relax with rectal distension.

13. *External sphincter contraction.* Observe contraction of the external sphincter with rectal distension, cough, or perineal pinprick.

14. *Rectal sensation.* Determine rectal sensation by inflating the rectal balloon with 50 cc of air and asking if the patient senses the distension. If the patient recognizes the sensation, decrease the distending volume in 5- to 10-cc increments to determine the *threshold* of rectal sensation. The threshold is the smallest volume of distension sensed. Also record the smallest volume that is associated with relaxation of the internal sphincter. The sensory threshold is influenced by the speed of inflation, so care should be taken to infuse at approximately the same rate each time. With rapid inflation, patients should perceive 10 cc or less.

Perfused and Solid-State System

The technique and equipment used for the perfused and solid-state system are similar to those used in esophageal manometry, as described in the chapter by Orlando, "Esophageal Manometry."

1. Calibrate the recording system according to the manufacturer's directions.

2. Inflate the rectal balloon with 50 cc of air for 30 sec. All the air should be recovered if the system is intact.

3. Lubricate the balloon.

4. The patient should lie on the left side, with knees bent. Carefully inspect the perineum and perianal area. Retract the buttocks to determine if the anal sphincter gapes. Check pinprick sensation bilaterally using the disposable needle and note the presence or absence of an anal wink. Ask the patient to perform the Valsalva maneuver to assess perineal descent.

Do a careful rectal examination. Ask the patient to contract the anus, noting the tone and response of the pelvic muscles.
5. Insert the catheter about 10 to 15 cm.
6. Use the continuous pull-out technique (or a mechanical pulling device) to identify the high-pressure zone. The pressure will rise as the recording ports enter the anal sphincter. Observe the location, length, and basal pressure of the sphincter zone. The pressure will fall to atmospheric as the ports are pulled past the sphincter. Stimulation of the sphincter will lead to spuriously high pressure readings. To obtain more accurate readings, first let the catheter remain undisturbed for several minutes to allow equilibration, then use a station pull-through approach to withdraw the catheter into the high-pressure zone. The catheter should be withdrawn 0.5 to 1 cm at a time with a 30-sec stabilization period at each station before the pressure is recorded.
7. Repeat the pull-through to confirm the pressure and location.
8. Insert the catheter into the high-pressure zone and distend the rectal balloon with 30 to 50 cc of air, to assess internal sphincter relaxation. If no reflex relaxation is seen, check the position of the catheter in the high-pressure zone and repeat.
9. *Rectal sensation.* Determine rectal sensation by inflating the rectal balloon with 50 cc of air and asking if the patient senses the distension. If the patient recognizes the sensation, decrease the distending volume in 5- to 10-cc increments to determine the *threshold* of rectal sensation. The threshold is the smallest volume of distension sensed. Also record the smallest volume that is associated with relaxation of the internal sphincter. The sensory threshold is influenced by the speed of inflation, so care should be taken to infuse at approximately the same rate each time. With rapid inflation, patients should perceive 10 cc or less.
10. To test for pelvic floor dyssynergia, position the catheter or EMG plug in the external sphincter and ask the patient to strain as if defecating. The normal response is a decrease in pressure.
11. Record the following pressures:
    a. *Maximal squeeze pressure.* Maximal squeeze pressure can be determined by positioning the catheter in the high-

pressure zone and asking the patient to maximally contract the sphincter. The pressure is the maximum absolute pressure recorded during the squeeze. Visual feedback of the recording can sometimes help the patient maximize the response. It may be necessary to move the catheter to find the position where the pressure is maximum.

b. *Squeeze increment.* This is the difference in pressure between the baseline and maximum pressure recorded.

c. *Rectal sensation and sensory threshold.* These are determined by inflating the rectal balloon with air as described above for the nonperfused system.

Postprocedure

1. Wash apparatus in warm, soapy water to remove stool and particulate matter.
2. Disinfect by soaking in glutaraldehyde.
3. Dry thoroughly.
4. Recalibrate the equipment if necessary.

Interpretation

Normal Internal Sphincter Response

In a normal response, the internal sphincter pressure will drop for up to 15 sec. The external sphincter should contract to preserve continence (Fig. 2). Most patients have relaxation down to a distending volume of 15 cc. Several repetitive rectal distensions in rapid succession produce a more pronounced relaxation of the internal sphincter. If the sphincter fails to relax, try rapid repetitive distension or try putting more air in the balloon. Also be sure that the patient is relaxed because strong contraction of the external sphincter, which surrounds the internal sphincter, can obscure the relaxation of the internal sphincter.

Normal Sphincter Pressures

Pressures can be determined by using the perfused system. Because of the broad range of normal pressures, the results must be

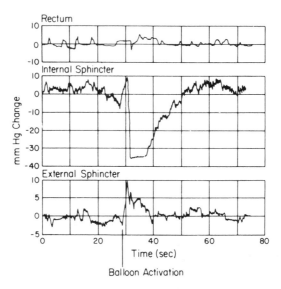

FIG. 2. The normal response to transient rectal distension is shown. The resting pressure of each balloon is assigned a value of zero with relaxation of the internal sphincter and contraction of the external sphincter.

interpreted in the context of the patient's history and complaints. In general, the normal resting basal pressure in adults is approximately 65 to 85 mm Hg above rectal intraluminal pressure using the continuous pull-through technique (1). Adults are generally able to generate squeeze pressures that are 50% to 100% above resting pressure. As a rule of thumb, a squeeze increment of 100 mm Hg or greater can be regarded as normal. Patients with pressures substantially below these values are at risk for incontinence, especially with liquid stools. This may be of prognostic significance in patients who have undergone an ileoanal pull-through.

Hirschsprung's Disease

In Hirschsprung's disease, the internal sphincter does not relax after transient rectal distension but, instead, may contract (Fig. 3) (2). The internal sphincter is invariably involved in Hirschsprung's disease. Rectal manometric studies may provide the

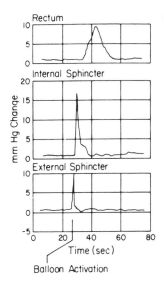

FIG. 3. Manometry response in a patient with Hirschsprung's disease. The internal sphincter contracts instead of relaxing following rectal distension. The external sphincter is normal, but a strong rectal contraction not seen in the normal follows contraction of the sphincters.

only means for establishing a diagnosis in short-segment Hirschsprung's disease.

Pelvic Floor Dyssynergia

In pelvic floor dyssynergia or anismus, the external sphincter and/or the puborectalis muscle contract instead of relaxing when the patient strains to defecate. This is most readily detected by positioning the perfused catheter or EMG plug in the high-pressure zone and asking the patient to strain.

Other Disorders

In scleroderma, the smooth internal sphincter muscle may fail to relax in response to rectal distension, whereas striated muscle is normal. In contrast, patients with polymyositis have impairment of the external sphincter but a normal internal sphincter (3). External sphincter dysfunction has been found in myotonic dystrophy, hypothyroidism, and myasthenia gravis. Patients with anal fissures may have a characteristic pattern of overshoot contraction of the internal sphincter following a normal relaxation.

Rectal manometry is not the first-line diagnostic study in any of these conditions.

Muscle Versus Nervous Dysfunction

The external sphincter response can be initiated by a number of stimuli such as voluntary effort, postural change, perianal scratch, rectal distension, and increased intraabdominal pressure (3). If the sphincter responds to any of these, the muscle is intact. If the sphincter fails to respond to all stimuli, there may be either muscle disease or a diffuse neurologic disorder. Following anal or rectal surgery the test may be performed to determine whether physiologic defects have been corrected (i.e., are within normal limits).

Biofeedback Therapy for Fecal Incontinence

Biofeedback refers to techniques in which information is provided to a patient about physiologic functions to gain control over these functions (4). Biofeedback has been applied quite successfully to the problem of fecal incontinence (5). There are a number of causes of fecal incontinence including anorectal surgery, spinal surgery or trauma, irritable bowel syndrome, rectal prolapse, diabetes, multiple sclerosis, scleroderma, and stroke. Continence has been restored with biofeedback in 70% to 83% of patients, often with one training session (4). The technique is simple, rapid, and without morbidity.

Most patients with impaired anal sphincters develop incontinence when they have diarrhea. Before embarking on a course of biofeedback, it is important to take a careful history to identify remedial causes of diarrhea. Lactose intolerance is a common cause of loose stools that is often not appreciated by the patient. Infection or irritable bowel should also be considered. The technique of biofeedback varies depending on the particular equipment used, and different centers use different protocols.

1. Perform standard manometry as described above. Either the perfused or the nonperfused apparatus may be used. Some prefer the nonperfused balloons for biofeedback because they

are easier to position in the sphincter and remain there. Anal plug electrodes are ideally suited to biofeedback.

2. Coach the patient to produce an upward deflection (increased pressure) on the manometric tracing of the external sphincter or an increase in EMG voltage.

3. In order to link the external sphincter contraction with rectal distension (and relaxation of the internal sphincter), ask the patient to momentarily (2 sec) contract the external sphincter whenever rectal distension is perceived. Distend the rectal balloon with 50 cc of air and offer praise if the external sphincter is appropriately contracted. Progressively decrease the volume of air distension until the sensation threshold is reached.

4. If the sensory threshold is high, progressively decrease the distending volume in the rectal balloon so that the patient senses smaller volumes and responds appropriately. Some incontinent patients will experience a delay in their perception of rectal distension (6). Some of them may be sensing the internal sphincter relaxing in response to the distending balloon rather than the distension itself. These patients should be conditioned to recognize the sensation of rectal distension and to eliminate the delay.

5. After conditioning with the recording in view, withhold visual feedback by blocking the patient's view of the tracing. Make sure that the patient performs the proper response without the visual feedback.

6. Perform distensions out of sight of the patient. Sessions may last 10 to 30 min. Stop when the patient becomes fatigued.

7. After the training session, instruct the patient to apply learned techniques consciously for 2 weeks whenever the sensation of rectal distension is felt. Indicate that the reflex will become automatic. For the first 6 to 8 weeks, the patient should practice momentary contractions four times a day, e.g., 25 squeezes each time.

9. Adding loperamide, 2 mg at bedtime, may be a useful adjunct to biofeedback. Loperamide increases anal canal pressure and attenuates the rectosphincteric relaxation reflex (7). It also decreases the frequency and looseness of stools. If constipation becomes a problem, the dose can be titrated, or

fiber supplements added. A bowel-training regimen designed to evacuate at a predictable time each day may be helpful to provide fewer opportunities for incontinence. In patients with fecal impaction as a contributing cause of fecal incontinence, bowel training should be tried prior to initiating biofeedback.

Biofeedback for Constipation

Biofeedback has also been used to treat constipation in adults with spastic pelvic floor syndrome (8) and in children with encopresis (9). The published experience on the use of biofeedback for constipation is not as extensive as for incontinence. There is considerable variation in reported techniques of biofeedback for constipation.

1. Perform standard manometry as described above. Either the perfused or nonperfused apparatus may be used. Some prefer the nonperfused balloons for biofeedback because they are easier to position in the sphincter and remain there. Anal plug electrodes are ideally suited to biofeedback for constipation.

2. Insert the sensing device into the anus and ask the patient to strain as during defecation. Normals will relax their perineum, reflected by a downward deflection in the manometric trace or a decrease in EMG voltage. Patients with constipation due to spastic pelvic floor will have a paradoxic pelvic floor contraction leading to obstructed defecation.

3. Instruct the patient to continue to strain but to try to develop maneuvers to relax the perineum during attempts to defecate. With successful relaxation, the sensing device may be evacuated.

4. A training session may consist of approximately 30 defecation trials over 45 min (9). Several sessions may be necessary to adequately reinforce the correct response.

5. Success is judged by improvement in bowel function. Some patients will learn to relax their pelvic floor in the manometry laboratory but will remain symptomatic.

REFERENCES

1. Wiley JW, Nostrant TT, Owyang C (1991): Evaluation of gastrointestinal motility: methodologic considerations. In: *Textbook of Gastroenterology*, edited by T Yamada, pp 2538–2561. JB Lippincott, Philadelphia.
2. Hirsh EH, Hodges KS, Hersh T, McGarity WC (1980): Anorectal manometry in the diagnosis of Hirschsprung's disease in adults. *Am J Gastroenterol* 74:258–260.
3. Schuster MM (1973): Diagnostic value of anal sphincter pressure measurements. *Hosp Pract* 8(4):115–117.
4. Marzuk PM (1985): Biofeedback for gastrointestinal disorders: a review of the literature. *Ann Intern Med* 103:240–244.
5. MacLeod JH (1987): Management of anal incontinence by biofeedback. *Gastroenterology* 93:291–294.
6. Buser WD, Miner PB (1986): Delayed rectal sensation with fecal incontinence: successful treatment using anorectal manometry. *Gastroenterology* 91:1186–1191.
7. Read NM, Read NW, Duthie HL (1980): The effect of loperamide on anal sphincter function. In: *Gastrointestinal Motility*, edited by J Christensen, pp 503–504. Raven Press, New York.
8. Bleijenberg G, Kuijpers HC (1987): Treatment of the spastic pelvic floor syndrome with biofeedback. *Dis Colon Rectum* 30:108–111.
9. Loening-Baucke V (1990): Modulation of abnormal defecation dynamics by biofeedback treatment in chronically constipated children with encopresis. *J Pediatr* 116:214–222.

10 / Secretin Injection Test for Diagnosis of Gastrinoma

John I. Wurzelmann and Robert S. Sandler

The diagnosis of gastrinoma (Zollinger-Ellison syndrome) can generally be made by demonstrating an elevation in serum gastrin and increased acid secretion in a patient with ulcer disease. If the fasting gastrin is greater than 1,000 pg/ml and gastric acid secretion is elevated, the patient almost certainly has a gastrinoma (1). However, there may be substantial overlap in serum gastrin and acid secretion between patients with gastrinoma and those with common peptic ulcer. Approximately 40% of patients with proven gastrinoma have fasting gastrins from 100 to 500 pg/ml, which is similar to the range seen in ulcer patients without gastrinomas (2). In order to increase the accuracy of diagnosis, a number of provocative tests have been devised (3). The secretin injection test is the most reliable and easiest to do (1).

Indication

Patients in whom the diagnosis of gastrinoma is suspected but not established or excluded.

Contraindications

None known.

Preparation

1. The patient should be fasting for 12 hr.
2. As antisecretory medications may affect serum gastrin, it is

reasonable to stop H_2 blockers 24 to 48 hr prior to the secretin test. If omeprazole is being used, it may be necessary to stop this medication 4 or 5 days in advance, treating the patient in the interim with an H_2 blocker.

Equipment

1. Large-bore (No. 18 or larger) intravenous catheter.
2. Seven small blood collection tubes, with labels to indicate when the samples are drawn.
3. Basin of ice.
4. Sterile three-way stopcock.
5. Intravenous (i.v.) tubing and bag of i.v. solution (D_5W).
6. Secretin-Ferring (Ferring Laboratories), 2.0 U/kg.
7. Eight 3-cc syringes.
8. Electric timer.
9. An assistant.

Procedure

1. Start a large-bore i.v. in an antecubital or other large vein.
2. Connect the intravenous catheter to the tubing via the three-way stopcock.
3. Clear the intravenous catheter of all i.v. solution by drawing a small quantity of blood and discarding it prior to collecting each sample.
4. Obtain baseline samples 10 min and 1 min before injection of secretin. Place samples on ice immediately.
5. Give 2.0 U/kg secretin by bolus injection over 30 sec.
6. Collect 3-cc samples at 2, 5, 10, 20, and 30 min (1).

Postprocedure

Remove the i.v.

Interpretation

More than 90% of patients with a gastrinoma will have an increase in gastrin, usually at 2 or 5 min (1). Because a small proportion of tests will only be positive within the first 2 min, care should be taken to obtain blood during this period (4). Although several criteria have been suggested (2), an absolute increase of 200 pg/ml is generally regarded as diagnostic (1). There may be occasional false-negatives using this criterion, and false-positives have been reported in persons with pentagastrin fast achlorhydria (5). For this reason, gastric acid secretion should be measured in hypergastrinemic patients before performing the secretin test. In normal individuals, those with duodenal ulcer disease, or those with antral G-cell hyperplasia, i.v. secretin either decreases or has no effect on serum gastrin levels. Some patients with duodenal ulcer and hypersecretion with no evidence of gastrinoma may have an increase in gastrin level after secretin (6), but the increase is less than 200 pg/ml.

REFERENCES

1. Jensen RT (1983): Differential diagnosis and provocative test. In: Jensen RT, moderator. Zollinger-Ellison syndrome: current concepts and management. *Ann Intern Med* 98:59–75.
2. Ippoliti AF (1977): Zollinger-Ellison syndrome: provocative diagnostic tests. *Ann Intern Med* 87: 787–788.
3. Wolfe MW, Jain DK, Edgerton JR (1985): Zollinger-Ellison syndrome associated with persistently normal fasting serum gastrin concentrations. *Ann Intern Med* 103:215–217.
4. Frucht H, Howard JM, Slaff JI, et al (1989): Secretin and calcium provocative tests in the Zollinger-Ellison syndrome: a prospective study. *Ann Intern Med* 111:713–722.
5. Feldman M, Schiller LR, Walsh JH, Fordtran JS, Richardson CT (1987): Positive intravenous secretin test in patients with achlorhydria related hypergastrinemia. *Gastroenterology* 93:59–62.
6. Malegelada J-R, Glanzman SL, Go VLW (1982): Laboratory diagnosis of gastrinoma. II. A prospective study of gastrin challenge tests. *Mayo Clin Proc* 57:219–226.

11 / Bentiromide Test for Diagnosis of Pancreatic Insufficiency

Ray L. James, Jr.

The bentiromide test is an orally administered noninvasive screening test for exocrine pancreatic insufficiency. Bentiromide (Chymex, Adria Laboratories) is cleaved by the pancreatic enzyme chymotrypsin liberating p-aminobenzoic acid (PABA), which is absorbed, conjugated by the liver, and excreted by the kidneys into the urine. The amount of PABA excreted can be determined by measuring the total urinary arylamine concentration. Since patients with exocrine pancreatic insufficiency have low levels of chymotrypsin available to cleave the bentiromide, less PABA is absorbed, and urine levels are decreased.

The bentiromide test has been shown to correlate with "invasive" tests of pancreatic exocrine function such as the secretin stimulation test or the Lundh meal test. Although the bentiromide test is less sensitive when pancreatic insufficiency is mild or moderate, it should be remembered that pancreatic exocrine function must be impaired by 90% or more before the disease is apparent (1).

Many variations of the standard bentiromide test have been suggested to improve the test results. These include measurement of serum PABA levels (1) or simultaneous administration of bentiromide and another marker excreted by the kidneys to generate a PABA excretion ratio (2,3). However, these variations are not routinely utilized at present and will not be described here.

Indications

1. To diagnose exocrine pancreatic insufficiency.
2. To monitor the adequacy of supplemental pancreatic enzyme therapy.

Contraindications

1. Patients with a known allergy to PABA.
2. Patients taking methotrexate, since PABA displaces methotrexate from binding sites.
3. Safe use during pregnancy, in nursing mothers, or in children under 6 yr old has *not* been established.

Preparation

1. Give nothing by mouth after midnight.
2. Discontinue 3 days before the test:
   a. Drugs that are metabolized to arylamines—

Acetaminophen	Chloramphenicol
Phenacetin	Procainamide
Benzocaine	Sulfonamides
Lidocaine	Thiazides
Procaine	

   b. Multivitamin or sunscreen preparations containing PABA.
   c. Prunes or cranberries from the diet.
3. Discontinue any pancreatic enzyme supplements for 5 days before the test.
4. Do not repeat the test for 7 days.

Procedure (4)

1. Have patient void immediately before drug administration.
2. For adults, administer orally 500 mg bentiromide (single-dose vial). For children, administer orally 14 mg/kg body weight.
3. Have the patient drink 250 mg water initially and at least another 250 mg within the first 2 hr of administration.
4. An additional 500 mg water or more may be given in hours 2 through 6 to stimulate urine flow.
5. Collect all urine for 6 hr, being sure that the patient voids at the 6-hr mark to complete the collection. Record the urine volume.
6. Refrigerate a 10-ml aliquot for analysis.

7. Submit the sample to a lab capable of performing the Smith modification of the Bratton-Marshall test for arylamines. (Check with your local laboratory about the availability of this assay before proceeding with the test.)

Postprocedure

Resume usual diet and medication.

Complications

There is the potential for allergic reactions to bentiromide or PABA, though this is rare. Diarrhea and headache are reported in less than 1 in 50 patients. Flatulence, nausea, vomiting, and weakness are reported in less than 1 in 160 patients.

Interpretation

1. The recovery of the PABA in the urine is determined by the following formula:

$$\% \text{ PABA recovered } - \frac{(\text{mg PABA/ml}) \ (V) \ (2.95)}{\text{mg bentiromide administered}}$$

   where mg PABA/ml is calculated by lab and corrected for dilution; V is urine volume from 6-hr collection; and 2.95 is the conversion factor. (Most labs will calculate the percent PABA recovered if the value for V and the bentiromide dose is supplied to them.)
2. A normal PABA excretion is greater than 50% to 57% (5). The smaller the value, the greater the likelihood of pancreatic insufficiency. Some patients with mild or even moderate pancreatic exocrine insufficiency may fall within the 50% to 75% range. All results less than 50% should be considered abnormal. A bar graph is available for further interpretation (Fig. 1).
3. False-positive tests (i.e., excretion <50%) may occur in patients with Billroth II gastrojejunostomy, small-intestine disease, liver disease, kidney disease, or diabetes mellitus.

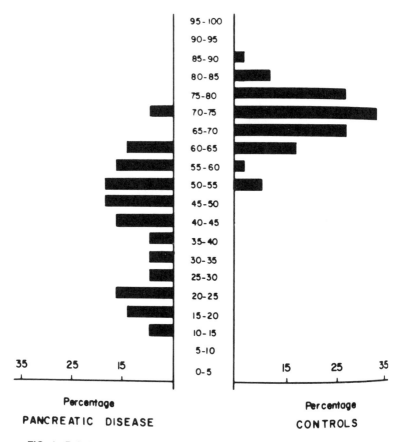

FIG. 1. Relative frequency distribution of urinary arylamines for patients with pancreatic disease and control subjects. Note overlap in 50% to 75% range (2).

4. The test does not differentiate between chronic pancreatitis, pancreatic cancer, or other potential causes of exocrine pancreatic insufficiency (6).

REFERENCES

1. Tanner AR, Robinson DP (1988): Pancreatic function testing: serum PABA measurement is a reliable and accurate measurement of exocrine function. *Gut* 29:1736–1740.
2. Hoek FJ, Van Den Bergh FAJTM, Klein Elhorst JT, Meijer JL, Timmer

E, Tytgat GNJ (1987): Improved specificity of the PABA test with p-aminosalicylic acid (PAS). *Gut* 28:468–473.

3. Puntis JWL, Berg JD, Buckley BM, Booth IW, McNeish AS (1988): Simplified oral pancreatic function test. *Arch Dis Child* 63:780–784.
4. Chymex (bentiromide): an oral screening test for exocrine pancreatic insufficiency. Adria Laboratories, Inc., Columbus Ohio 43215.
5. Toskes PP (1983): Bentiromide as a test of exocrine pancreatic function in adult patients with pancreatic exocrine insufficiency: determination of appropriate dose and urinary collection interval. *Gastroenterology* 85:565–569.
6. Niederau C, Grendell JH (1985): Diagnosis of chronic pancreatitis. *Gastroenterology* 88:1973–1995.

12 / Abdominal Paracentesis

Henry R. Lesesne

Aspiration and examination of peritoneal fluid has been an important diagnostic procedure for many years in the differential diagnosis of ascites and acute abdomen and in the evaluation of blunt trauma to the abdomen. Recently, therapeutic large-volume paracentesis has gained acceptance (1).

Indications

1. Evaluation and therapy of ascites.
2. Detection of perforated viscus in a patient with an acute abdomen or following blunt trauma to the abdomen.

Contraindications

1. Disorders of blood coagulation:
   a. Prothrombin time >5 sec of control.
   b. Platelet count <50,000/mm^3.
2. Intestinal obstruction.
3. Infection of the abdominal wall.
4. Relative contraindications:
   a. Poor patient cooperation.
   b. History of multiple abdominal surgeries.

Preparation of Patient

1. Obtain hematocrit, prothrombin time, and platelet count at least 48 hr prior to procedure.
2. Explain the risks, benefits, and details of the procedure to the patient.
3. Obtain written consent.

Equipment

1. Sterile gloves.
2. Povidone-iodine (Betadine) and alcohol; sterile gauze.
3. Draping towels.
4. Local anesthetic (lidocaine, 1%) and needles.
5. Syringes: 10 cc × 2, 50 cc × 2.
6. Paracentesis needles:
   a. No. 16, 18, 20 gauge.
   b. Spinal needle (No. 18, 20 gauge) for obese patients.
7. Sterile specimen tubes.
8. If infection suspected, blood culture bottles for bedside inoculation (2).

Procedure

Diagnostic Paracentesis

1. Have patient empty bladder.
2. Position the patient in the bed with the head elevated 45° to 90°. This allows fluid to accumulate in lower abdomen. (If there is a small volume of ascitic fluid, the patient can be asked to assume the knee-hand position on the side of the bed with the physician working from below.)
3. Identify the point of aspiration: in the midline midway between the umbilicus and pubic bone (Fig. 1). If scars from previous surgeries are present, choose the right or left lower quadrant lateral to the rectus muscles.
4. Put on sterile gloves.
5. Sterilize the site with povidone-iodine and then alcohol.
6. Place sterile draping towels.
7. Inject lidocaine down to and including the peritoneum.
8. Attach a No. 18 gauge needle (spinal needle for obese patients) to a 10-cc syringe and insert this into the peritoneal cavity and inject 5 cc air.
9. Gently aspirate 10 cc fluid, and then attach 50-cc syringe and aspirate further quantities of fluid as needed for predetermined analysis (usually 100–200 cc).
10. If no fluid returns after several attempts, ultrasound-directed aspiration should be used.

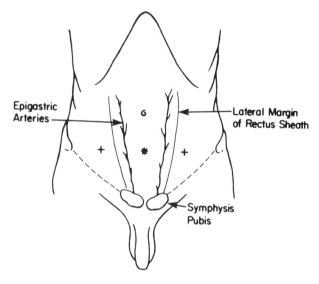

FIG. 1. Various sites of paracentesis: (*) preferred; (+) secondary.

11. Remove the needle and place an adhesive bandage (Band-Aid) or pressure dressing over the site. The patient may resume normal activities.

Therapeutic Paracentesis

Removal of large amounts (>1 liter) of ascitic fluid was commonplace decades ago, but fell into disuse with the advent of potent diuretics unless respiratory difficulty occurred from a tense abdomen. Recent studies showing the safety and patient acceptance of large-volume paracentesis have resulted in the return of this therapeutic procedure in massive ascites (1,3).

1. Equipment:
    a. Thoracentesis tray with thoracentesis catheter (7 in. long, with No. 14 gauge × 2-in. needle) (4).
    b. 1-liter vacuum bottles (× 5).
2. Prepare the patient as in diagnostic paracentesis.
3. Place intravenous heparin lock for albumin infusion (10 g for each liter removed).

4. Using the thoracentesis catheter attached to a 10-cc syringe, slowly advance needle and catheter into peritoneal cavity and aspirate fluid.
5. Attach tubing to catheter and insert into 1-liter vacuum bottle.
6. Aspirate 4 to 6 liters of ascitic fluid using this apparatus over 30 to 60 min.
7. Remove the catheter and place bandage or absorbable suture at puncture site. Pressure bandage may be applied.
8. Monitor vital signs hourly for 2 to 4 hr post procedure.
9. Repeat large-volume paracentesis can be performed on successive days if patient's hemodynamic status and renal function remain stable.
10. Send sample of fluid from each paracentesis for white blood cell count and differential to detect onset of unsuspected bacterial peritonitis.

Analysis of Fluid

The analysis of the aspirated fluid will be determined by the individual patient and his or her diagnosis. Routine tests employed include the following:

1. Total protein and albumin (5).
2. Red and white blood cell count.
3. Gram and acid–fast bacillus (AFB) stains.
4. Amylase.
5. Culture (bacterial, AFB, fungal, viral).
6. Cytology (at last 50 cc).
7. Other chemistries as indicated: CEA, lactate dehydrogenase, triglyceride, cholesterol, etc.

Complications

The incidence of serious complications from paracentesis is rare, as recently described in a prospective study by Runyon (6). Of 229 procedures, 1 patient had transfusion-requiring abdominal wall hematomas, and 2 patients had non–transfusion-requiring hematomas. No bacterial peritonitis or death occurred. An earlier study suggested a higher complication rate (7/242) in patients with cirrhosis (7).

REFERENCES

1. Kellerman PS, Linas SL (1990): Large-volume paracentesis in the treatment of ascites. *Ann Intern Med* 112:889–890.
2. Runyon BA, Umland ET, Merlin T (1987): Inoculation of blood culture bottles with ascitic fluid. Improved detection of spontaneous bacterial peritonitis. *Arch Intern Med* 147:73–75.
3. Salerno F, Badalamenti S, Incerti P, et al (1987): Repeated paracentesis and i.v. albumin infusion to treat "tense" ascites in cirrhotic patients. A safe alternative therapy. *J Hepatol* 5:102–108.
4. Pharmaseal. Thorancentesis Tray. American Pharmaseal Company, Valencia, California 91355-8900.
5. Rector WG Jr, Reynolds TB (1984): Superiority of serum-ascites albumin difference over ascites total protein concentration in separation of "transudative" and "exudative" ascites. *Am J Med* 77:83–85.
6. Runyon BA (1986): Paracentesis of ascitic fluid. A safe procedure. *Arch Intern Med* 146:2259–2261.
7. Mallory A, Schaefer JW (1978): Complications of diagnostic paracentesis in patients with liver disease. *JAMA* 239:628–630.

13 / Percutaneous Peritoneal Biopsy

Henry R. Lesesne

Needle biopsy of the peritoneum is a useful adjunct to the evaluation of a patient with unexplained ascites (1,2). Percutaneous biopsy using the Cope needle is simple and inexpensive. At times, direct peritoneal biopsy during peritoneoscopy is indicated. (Most of the information in the chapter by Lesesne, "Abdominal Paracentesis," applies here.) The following specifically relates to the percutaneous biopsy of the peritoneum using the Cope needle.

Indications

Peritoneal biopsy should be considered to rule out tuberculosis, fungal infection, and metastatic carcinoma in a patient with exudative ascites, particularly when bacterial cultures and cytology are negative.

Contraindications

1. Prothrombin time >3 sec.
2. Platelets, <50,000/mm^3.
3. Portal hypertension with evidence of collateral circulation.

Equipment

1. Equipment used in therapeutic paracentesis (see chapter by Lesesne, "Abdominal Paracentesis").
2. Cope needle (trocar, biopsy shaft, and snare).
3. Formalin solution for fixation of tissue.

Preparation

See chapter by Lesesne, "Abdominal Paracentesis."

Procedure

1. Prepare the patient and give local anesthetic as described.
2. Do not attempt this procedure if ascitic fluid is not easily aspirated with the anesthetic needle.
3. Make a 2-mm skin incision at the biopsy site. Levine (1) prefers biopsying in the left lower quadrant (see Fig. 1 in the chapter by Lesesne, "Abdominal Paracentesis").
4. Introduce the biopsy shaft and trocar into the peritoneal cavity.
5. Have the assistant apply pressure to the contralateral side of the abdomen to create a large cushion of fluid in the operating area.
6. If fluid is needed for further examination, remove the trocar and aspirate.
7. Introduce the snare (needle) attached to a syringe through the biopsy shaft and withdraw the snare until it engages the peritoneum.
8. Complete the biopsy by rotating the biopsy shaft forward over the snare.
9. Remove the snare, but not the shaft.
10. Fix the tissue in formalin or place in sterile container with sterile saline for culture.
11. Repeat the procedure three or four times with the tip of the snare in different directions to obtain several samples.
12. Close the incision with absorbable sutures and apply a pressure dressing.
13. Send the biopsy specimens in the labeled formalin jar to the laboratory.

Postprocedure

1. Monitor vital signs for 6 hr (q.1 hr).
2. Keep the patient at bed rest for 6 hr.

REFERENCES

1. Levine H (1967): Needle biopsy of peritoneum in exudative ascites. *Arch Intern Med* 120:542–545.
2. Jenkins PF, Ward MJ (1980): The role of peritoneal biopsy in the diagnosis of ascites. *Postgrad Med J* 56:702–703.

14 / Percutaneous Liver Biopsy

Henry R. Lesesne

Percutaneous liver biopsy is a widely used, well-established, and generally safe procedure that is useful and important in the evaluation and management of patients with many liver disorders (1). Because it is a potentially hazardous, invasive procedure, it should be undertaken only after initial noninvasive studies of liver disease have been unproductive or suggest a need for examination of liver tissue. Outpatient liver biopsy can be considered if appropriate facilities are available (2). Difficult cases (obesity, small liver, unsuccessful blind biopsy) can be aided by ultrasonic or computed tomography (CT) localization (3). For focal lesions of the liver (found not to be cystic), fine-needle aspiration biopsy under radiologic direction may be the first invasive procedure to consider, especially if malignancy is suspected (4). When tense ascites or severe coagulation defects are present, transvenous needle biopsy may be considered (5).

Indications

1. To diagnose suspected primary liver disease or unexplained hepatomegaly.
2. To assess the course of certain liver diseases (e.g., chronic active hepatitis) and response to therapy.
3. To confirm the presence of malignant disease.
4. To assist in the diagnosis and staging of lymphomas.
5. To assist in the diagnoses of metabolic disease (e.g., glycogen storage disease), multisystem disease (e.g., sarcoidosis, tuberculosis, or hemochromatosis), or pyrexia of unknown origin. (Biopsy specimens may be cultured and stained for specific organisms.)

6. To assess the effect of hepatotoxic drugs (e.g., methotrexate in treatment of psoriasis).

Contraindications

1. Uncooperative patient.
2. Abnormal clotting parameters:
   a. Prothrombin time (PT) >3 sec of control.
   b. Partial thromboplastin time (PTT) >20 sec of control.
   c. Thrombin clotting time (TCT) >4 to 5 sec of control.
   d. Platelet count <75,000/mm^3.
   e. Prolonged bleeding time (>10 min).
3. Severe anemia, hematocrit (Hct) <25%.
4. Local infection:
   a. Infected pleural effusion.
   b. Peritonitis (ascites should be cultured prior to biopsy).
5. Massive, tense ascites.
6. High-grade extrahepatic obstructive jaundice.
7. Severe uremia (BUN >50).

Preparation

The following guidelines are for *inpatient liver biopsy* but can be modified for outpatients as well.

To be done prior to the procedure:

1. Prebiopsy checklist:
   a. Check patient's general condition and cooperation.
   b. Obtain Hct, BUN, PT, PTT, TCT within 48 hr of biopsy.
   c. Obtain bleeding time.
   d. Review chest film (look for pleural effusion or, rarely, bowel under right diaphragm).
   e. Review liver imaging (CT, liver scan) if obtained.
   f. Send clot to blood bank: "Type and screen—liver biopsy tomorrow."
2. Explain the procedure including benefits, risks, and alternatives; have consent form signed and witnessed.
3. Write prebiopsy note to include:
   a. Statement of indication for liver biopsy.

b. Statement of any contraindications to biopsy. Explain if any relative contraindications exist and note precautions that will be taken.
4. Write orders for procedure:
   a. Nothing by mouth after midnight.
   b. The following to be at bedside in the morning:
      i. Liver biopsy tray.
      ii. Two pairs of gloves size _____.
      iii. Povidone-iodine (Betadine), alcohol, and 1% lidocaine.
      iv. Six 5-cc vials sterile saline.
      v. Sterile bottles for cytology and culture specimens.
      vi. Adhesive bandage (Band-Aid).
      vii. 10% Formalin solution for fixation of specimen.
   c. To empty the gallbladder, have the patient drink a carton of milk 1 hr before procedure.
   d. Heparin lock for intravenous access is prudent for patients with anemia, mild coagulation defects, and any cardiopulmonary instability.

The liver biopsy tray should include the following (see Preparation, item 4,b):

1. Klatskin or Menghini liver biopsy needle (No. 16 gauge).
2. Petri dish.
3. No. 11 blade and holder.
4. Gauze.
5. Forceps.
6. Syringes (10 cc × 2).
7. Punch, to make hole in skin to allow needle to pass.
8. Spinal needle (No. 22 gauge) to determine depth of diaphragm from skin for obese patients.
9. Sterile towels.

Procedure (1,6)

Position patient near edge of bed with right arm under the head and left arm by left side.

Identify Site for Liver Biopsy (Fig. 1)

1. Slightly posterior to midaxillary line.
2. Two finger-breadths below the upper border of hepatic dullness or midway between the upper and lower borders of hepatic dullness.
3. Above the bottom rib of the intercostal space.

Teach patient to hold his or her breath at end-expiration while using your finger to simulate the needle stick.

Sterilize Biopsy Area

1. Put on gown, mask, and eye guards.
2. Wash hands and put on sterile gloves.
3. Cleanse the area thoroughly with Betadine or other cleansing solution. Begin at the biopsy site and wash with an expanding circular motion.
4. Repeat in the same manner using alcohol.
5. Drape the patient with sterile towels.

Prepare Site for Biopsy

1. Infiltrate needle tract through skin, subcutaneous tissue, and diaphragm with 1% lidocaine. The tract should be horizontal

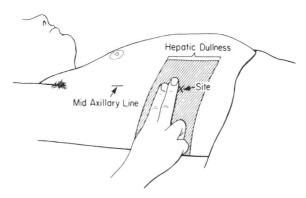

FIG. 1. Percutaneous liver biopsy.

to the bed and about 5° off the perpendicular in the direction of the xiphoid.

2. With the punch (or No. 11 blade), make a small incision in the skin (this will allow easy passage of the liver biopsy needle).

3. In obese patients with rib spaces that are difficult to palpate, use the spinal needle to find the depth of the diaphragm:
   a. Slowly insert needle into the tract.
   b. Every 5 mm, ask the patient to breathe.
   c. You are in the diaphragm when the needle head moves downward toward the patient's feet.
   d. You are in the liver when the needle head moves upward toward the patient's head. Note the distance from the skin to the diaphragm (approximately 1–2 cm) for placement of liver biopsy needle.

Perform Liver Biopsy

1. Attach the liver biopsy needle to a 10-cc syringe filled with saline fluid.

2. Insert the liver biopsy needle to the diaphragm. Be certain you are past the rib so that it will not be hit during the actual biopsy.

3. Flush 1 cc saline fluid through needle to clear it of skin or fat.

4. Ask patient to take in a breath, blow it all out, and hold in end-expiration.

5. Grasp the needle with your left hand 3.0 cm from skin. This is your guard.

6. With your right hand, produce negative pressure by withdrawing syringe plunger 1 to 2 cc (for cirrhosis, use 3-cc suction).

7. In one motion, push syringe and needle in 3.0 cm (to finger guard) and come out quickly. Suction should be maintained at all times. This "1-sec technique" will allow the liver specimen to be aspirated into the saline fluid–filled syringe.

8. If bleeding occurs, apply direct pressure to puncture site with sterile gauze.

9. At least 2.5 cm of liver tissue is needed for examination. A

second or third biopsy should be performed for more tissue, and especially to minimize sampling error (e.g., chronic hepatitis).

Fix Liver Specimens

1. Express 1 cc of fluid into Petri dish through the needle to remove any tissue remaining in needle.
2. Remove the syringe plunger and allow the tissue specimen and saline fluid in the syringe to flow into the Petri dish.
3. Decant the excess saline fluid from the Petri dish without disturbing the liver specimen.
4. Pour the formalin solution into the Petri dish to fix the specimen.

Have the patient slowly turn onto the right side. The patient should be able to move his or her arms and legs while keeping constant body pressure on the biopsy site for 2 hr. The next 10 to 12 hr will be spent at bed rest.

Cytology

1. Inject fluid aspirated from the Petri dish into the sterile specimen bottle.
2. Send fluid for cytology.

Culture[1]

1. Leave a small amount of saline fluid in sterile specimen bottle along with a small piece of liver (0.5–1.0 cm).
2. Cover sterile bottle.
3. Send sterile bottle to microbiology lab for routine, acid–fast bacillus (AFB), and fungal cultures as needed.
4. If viral cultures desired, place small piece of liver in appropriate medium at the bedside.

---

[1]Culture specimens should be obtained *prior* to formalin fixation of the specimens.

Histopathology

1. Return the liver specimen and formalin to the specimen bottle.
2. Send to histopathology lab, noting the time the specimen was fixed.

Postprocedure

Procedure Note

Write procedure note. Include what was done, location of the biopsy site, how many "passes" were made, where the specimens were sent, and a description of the gross specimen.

Post–Liver Biopsy Orders

Write post–liver biopsy orders. Suggested format:

1. Strict bed rest for 10 hr; first 2 hr on right side. Patient may sit up after 4 hr.
2. Blood pressure, pulse: every 15 min $\times$ 2 hr; every 30 min $\times$ 2 hr; every 1 hr $\times$ 6 hr.
3. Notify physician on call if blood pressure <90/60 mm Hg, pulse >110 bpm, or severe pain experienced.
4. Diet: full liquids for 6 hr, then resume regular diet.
5. Obtain venous Hct in 6 hr.

Post–Liver Biopsy Note

Write a post–liver biopsy note (4 and 10 hr post biopsy):

1. Statement of condition of patient and any complications noted.
2. If discharged, give patient warning signs to call immediately (return of severe pain, dizziness, fever, etc.).

Complications (1,7)

Pain over the liver and right shoulder occur in 5% to 10% of patients but rarely require analgesia. Major complications (intraabdominal hemorrhage, bile peritonitis, and perforation of gall-bladder or colon) are very rare and often respond to conservative measures with close observation coupled with surgical consultation.

REFERENCES

1. Maddrey WC (1991): Needle biopsy of the liver. In: *George D. Zuidema's Shackelford's Surgery of the Alimentary Tract, Vol III*, edited by G Turcotte, pp 292–295. WB Saunders Company, Philadelphia.
2. Westaby D, Macdougall BRD, Williams R (1980): Liver biopsy as a day-case procedure—selection and complications in 200 consecutive patients. *Br Med J* 281:1331–1332.
3. Bjork JT, Foley WD, Varma RR (1981): Percutaneous liver biopsy in difficult cases simplified by CT or ultrasound localization. *Dig Dis Sci* 26:146–148.
4. Buscarini L, Fornari F, Bolondi L, et al (1990): Ultrasound-guided fine-needle biopsy of focal liver lesions: techniques, diagnostic accuracy and complications. *J Hepatol* 11:344–348.
5. Lebrec D, Goldfarb G, Degott C, Rueff B, Benhamou JP (1982): Trans-venous liver biopsy. *Gastroenterology* 83:338–340.
6. Ishak KG, Schiff ER, Schiff L (1987): Needle biopsy of the liver. In: *Diseases of the Liver*, edited by L Schiff, ER Schiff, pp 399–441. JB Lippincott Company, Philadelphia.
7. Perrault J, McGill DB, Ott BJ, Taylor WF (1978): Liver biopsy: complications in 1000 inpatients and outpatients. *Gastroenterology* 74:103–106.

15 / Diagnostic Peritoneoscopy (Laparoscopy)

Henry R. Lesesne

Until recently, peritoneoscopy has been of limited use in internal medicine. It is now considered one of the most reliable techniques available for closing the gap between clinical evaluation and surgical exploration (1). Surgeons have recently expanded on the use of this technique by introducing laparoscopic cholecystectomy (2). This chapter describes diagnostic laparoscopy only.

Indications

1. Guided liver biopsy under direct visualization.
2. Guided biopsies of the peritoneum to aid in the evaluation of ascites.
3. Assessing operability among patients with proven carcinoma.
4. Staging of lymphomas.
5. Evaluation of intraabdominal masses.
6. Evaluation of suspected pelvic pathology.
7. Evaluation of patients with acute abdominal trauma.

Contraindications

1. Poor patient cooperation (general anesthesia may be considered).
2. Disorders of blood coagulation:
   a. Prothrombin time (PT) >3 sec of control.
   b. Partial thromboplastin time (PTT) >20 sec of control.
   c. Thrombin clotting time (TCT) >4 to 5 sec of control.
   d. Platelet count <100,000/mm^3.
   e. Bleeding time >10 min.

3. Hematocrit (Hct) <30%.
4. Peritonitis.
5. Intestinal obstruction.
6. Infection of abdominal wall.
7. Relative contraindications:
   a. Severe cardiac or pulmonary disease.
   b. Large abdominal hernias.
   c. History of multiple abdominal surgeries (adhesions will decrease visualization and increase risk of perforation).

Preparation of Patient

1. X-ray and laboratory studies:
   a. Obtain Hct, BUN, PT, PTT, TCT, and bleeding time, at least 48 hr prior to procedure.
   b. Obtain and review chest X-ray, kidney-ureter-bladder (KUB) film, and EKG.
   c. Type and cross for 2 U of whole blood or packed red cells.
   d. Culture ascitic fluid.
   e. Review liver scan and/or CT scan (if available).
2. Explain the risks, benefits, and details of the procedure to the patient.
3. Have patient sign informed consent.
4. Write a preperitoneoscopy note to include:
   a. Statement of indication for procedure.
   b. Statement that there are no contraindications, or explanation of the relative contraindications, detailing precautions to be taken.
   c. Orders:
      i. Give nothing by mouth following midnight.
      ii. Begin intravenous fluids (D_5W) at 8 A.M.
      iii. Give Fleet enema at 8 A.M.
      iv. On call to procedure, have patient empty bladder.
      v. Perform abdominal shave, if there is excessive hair growth around the umbilicus.

Equipment[1]

1. Fiberoptic projector with light-transmitting cable.
2. Nitrous oxide (N_2O) automatic insufflator with tubing.
3. Verres cannula for pneumoperitoneum.
4. Operating peritoneoscope and accessory instruments:
   a. Cannula with trumpet valve and trocar.
   b. Operating scope.
   c. Biopsy forceps.
   d. Liver biopsy needle for scope.
5. Second puncture instrument with biopsy forceps.
6. Standard liver biopsy tray to be used for guided liver biopsy using the percutaneous approach.
7. Accessories for procedure:
   a. Draping towels ($\times$ 6).
   b. Povidone-iodine (Betadine) and alcohol.
   c. Syringes: 10 cc $\times$ 3 to 4; 50 cc $\times$ 1.
   d. Needles for local anesthetic.
   e. Bard-Parker blade (No. 11).
   f. Absorbable suture; Steri-Strips.
   g. Local anesthetic [bupivacaine hydrochloride (Marcaine) or lidocaine hydrochloride (Xylocaine), 1%].
   h. Hemostats ($\times$ 6); forceps ($\times$ 2).
   i. Scissors.
   j. Gauze sponges.

Procedure

Peritoneoscopy may be performed in a well-equipped endoscopy suite that contains resuscitation equipment. Physician trainees should learn this procedure in the operating room with an experienced peritoneoscopist in attendance. An assistant is needed to obtain biopsy specimens. A surgeon should be on call or available for any complications.

---

[1]Recommended peritoneoscopy equipment and accessories are made by American Cystoscope Makers, Inc.; Eder Instrument Company; Storz Instrument Company; and Richard Wolf Instrument Company.

1. With patient supine, infuse meperidine, 25 to 50 mg, slowly (naloxone should be available for respiratory depression); then infuse diazepam (1 mg/min) until slurred speech or horizontal nystagmus occurs.
2. Put on a mask and surgical gown and hand scrub for 5 min. Put on sterile gloves.
3. Sterilize the abdomen with diluted povidone-iodine from nipples to pubis with the center of sterilization around umbilicus. (This large area allows for a second puncture during procedure.)
4. Inject local anesthetic down to and including the peritoneum. The sites for insertion of instrument are shown in Figure 1. Avoid areas of previous surgery, enlarged organs, the falciform ligament, and the epigastric vessels. If cirrhosis is present, collateral veins may form around the umbilicus— insertion should be done with caution and possibly in the left upper quadrant in such circumstances.
5. Make a 5-mm horizontal incision with the Bard-Parker blade and insert the Verres (pneumoperitoneum) needle into the peritoneum, with the patient tensing his or her abdomen with a Valsalva maneuver.
6. Infuse N_2O (2–3 liters) and remove the Verres needle.
7. Extend the incision to about 1.0 to 1.5 cm (enough to allow cannula with trocar to pass through the skin without causing N_2O leakage).
8. Insert the cannula with trocar during a Valsalva maneuver.
9. Remove the trocar. Place the peritoneoscope in the cannula and pass it into the peritoneum under direct visualization.
10. Systematically inspect the abdominal contents, noting the appearance of the peritoneum, pelvic organs, intestine, mesentery, liver, spleen, and diaphragm.
11. Biopsy procedures (to be done only after full inspection of the abdomen):
    a. *Liver*. The liver can be biopsied through the operating scope with either the special liver biopsy needle or forceps (for accessible, focal lesions). Biopsy can also be performed using the percutaneous liver biopsy needle inserted over the liver with guidance by the peritoneoscopist. Likewise, the second puncture instrument can be in-

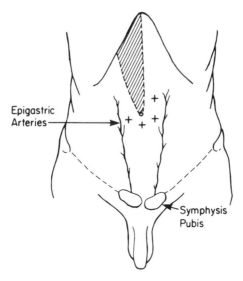

FIG. 1. Various sites for insertion of peritoneoscope; (*shaded area*) falciform ligament.

serted over the liver, and focal lesions biopsied with forceps. Local anesthetic should be sprayed over the liver (or peritoneum) using tubing inserted through the peritoneoscope prior to biopsy.

b. *Peritoneum.* Guided peritoneal biopsy can be done with the scope forceps or with the second puncture instrument and forceps.

c. *Other structures.* Mass lesions involving other organs (mesentery, spleen, stomach wall, pancreas) can be biopsied with forceps, being careful not to biopsy highly vascular lesions or pulsating masses.

12. Aspirate ascitic fluid for culture and cytologies as needed.

13. To complete the procedure:

a. Remove the scope. Allow N_2O to escape by asking the patient to do several Valsalva maneuvers.

b. Remove the cannula.

c. Close the incision with two to four subcutaneous absorbable sutures. Cover with an adhesive bandage (Band-Aid). Steri-Strips or suture may be used to close second puncture instrument incision.

14. Processing of biopsy material. The biopsy material should be handled as explained under Procedure in the chapter "Percutaneous Liver Biopsy" by Lesesne.

Postperitoneoscopy Procedure

1. The patient should be returned to the recovery room with orders written, as under Postprocedure in "Percutaneous Liver Biopsy" by Lesesne. The dictated operative note should include:
   a. Preoperative diagnosis.
   b. Postoperative diagnosis and findings.
   c. Operation.
   d. Names of attending physician and assistants.
   e. Anesthesia used.
   f. Specimens (pathology, cytology) taken.
   g. Cultures done.
   h. Estimated blood loss.
   (A summary of these findings should be recorded in the chart.)
2. The physician should evaluate the patient at 4 and 8 hr post procedure, assessing for signs of active bleeding or peritonitis and recording any notable findings. (*Note.* A small amount of N_2O may remain and cause minimal abdominal pain. Mild analgesia may be used.)
3. The patient may be discharged 8 hr following procedure if stable.

Equipment Sterilization

Sterilization of instruments and accessories is safely carried out by the ethylene oxide method available in most hospitals. Cold sterilization can also be done using a solution such as 2% glutaraldehyde. The instrument should soak for at least 20 min (1).

Complications

Complications of peritoneoscopy are infrequent but can be major, requiring surgery. One prospective study covering 7 years and 603 laparoscopies found 31 (5.1%) minor complications and 14 (2.3%) major complications requiring surgery or transfusion (hemorrhage and perforation of the colon) (4).

REFERENCES

1. Boyce WH Jr (1987): Laparoscopy. In: *Diseases of the Liver*, edited by L Schiff, ER Schiff, pp 443–456. JB Lippincott Company, Philadelphia.
2. Salky BA (1990): *Laparoscopy for Surgeons*. Igaku-Shoin, New York.
3. Beck K (1982): *Color Atlas of Laparoscopy*. WB Saunders Company, Philadelphia.
4. Kane MG, Krejs GJ (1984): Complications of diagnostic laparoscopy in Dallas: a 7-year prospective study. *Gastrointest Endosc* 30:237–240.

16 / Percutaneous Transhepatic Cholangiography

Kim L. Isaacs and Sidney L. Levinson

Percutaneous transhepatic cholangiography (PTC) is a diagnostic modality useful in the evaluation of the patient with suspected obstructive jaundice. When noninvasive examinations suggest biliary obstruction, a PTC or endoscopic retrograde cholangiogram (ERC) is the next diagnostic step. These studies delineate changes in the extrahepatic and intrahepatic biliary tree including strictures, tumor, and retained gallstones. In most cases PTC and ERC provide similar information about the bile duct disease (1,2). PTC is especially helpful in cases where ERC has failed or provided unclear information, in patients who have had previous bile duct or bowel surgery making the biliary system inaccessible to the duodenoscope, in cases where the biliary tree proximal to an obstruction is not well visualized by ERC, and in patients who are unable to tolerate ERC (1). When bile ducts are dilated, the diagnostic yield of PTC approaches 100% and is usually well tolerated (3,5).

Indications

1. Diagnosis of obstructive jaundice.
2. Establishment of anatomic detail of intrahepatic and extrahepatic bile ducts.
3. Identification of stones, parasites, bifurcation tumors, and other space-occupying lesions.
4. Highlighting changes of the biliary tree in pancreatic disease (e.g., chronic pancreatitis, pancreatic carcinoma).

116

Contraindications

Absolute

1. Bleeding abnormalities [see chapter by Lesesne, "Diagnostic Peritoneoscopy (Laparoscopy)"].
2. Active sepsis, peritonitis, or cellulitis of the abdominal wall.
3. Sensitivity to contrast media.
4. Suspicion of cystic echinococcal disease or hypervascular tumor of the liver (1).

Relative

1. High or continuous fever.
2. Moderate to severe anemia.
3. Ascites.
4. Metastatic cancer involving the liver.

Preparation

Antibiotics (6,7)

See chapter by Isaacs, "Medications in the GI Procedure Unit."

Coagulation Parameters

Check coagulation parameters and institute measures to correct abnormalities (vitamin K, cessation of aspirin several days to weeks prior to procedure, administration of plasma or factor concentrates in patients with documented factor deficiencies).

Equipment

1. Fluoroscopy suite. Emergency facilities to manage dye reactions or other complications.
2. No. 22 gauge needle, 15 cm long, with an inner fitting stylet and a short 30° noncutting bevel (Chiba needle).
3. Povidone-iodine solution, 1% injectable lidocaine, syringes,

No. 22 and 25 gauge needles, No. 11 blade, and sterile drapes for preparation of the needle stick site.

4. Contrast medium (iopromide, 300 mg Iodine/ml).
5. Intravenous midazolam or other benzodiazepine for sedation. Narcotics and/or antiemetics may also be used.

Procedure (1,3–5,8,9)

1. Place the patient supine on the fluoroscopy table; support the head with the patient's right arm.
2. Drape the lower right lateral chest wall and prepare with povidone-iodine solution.
3. Select the area of puncture in the eighth or ninth intercostal space (based on liver size). This is just below the costophrenic angle, at or just anterior to the midaxillary line (10–13 cm off the table). The lateral approach provides a longer tract for tamponade of blood and bile.
4. Locally infiltrate the area with lidocaine. Make a 3-mm stab with a surgical blade.
5. Have the patient hold his or her breath at end-expiration and pass the needle, with the stylet in place, horizontal to the table. *The pass is made under fluoroscopic control, aimed toward a point just to the left of the dome of the right diaphragm, avoiding the confluence of the main hepatic ducts* (Fig. 1). The border of the vertebral bodies is used as an endpoint for the pass; however, some authors do not rely on the often inconstant relationships of the liver, lung, and vertebrae (9).
6. Remove the stylet and attach a syringe filled with contrast.
7. With the patient resuming shallow respirations, withdraw the needle slowly, several millimeters at a time. Apply gentle pressure to the plunger while injecting 0.1 to 1.0 ml of contrast. The pattern of contrast seen on fluoroscopy will determine a successful injection. Slow hepatofugal flow in linear structures, which may be persistent, particularly with obstruction, denotes bile ducts. Other possible patterns include the following:
   a. An indistinct blush usually denotes liver parenchyma.

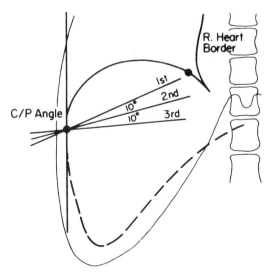

FIG. 1. Insertion of Chiba needle.

b. Serpiginous thin vessels flowing to the liver hilum are lymph vessels.

c. A stellate network of channels carrying contrast rapidly to the liver hilum and on to the right atrium denotes blood vessels.

8. Fill the ducts with a minimum of contrast. Aspiration of bile is usually not necessary. However, if dilated ducts are encountered, bile is remove in 30- to 100-cc amounts and contrast is given milliliter for milliliter. Take care to avoid overdistension of the ducts. Sepsis is more likely to occur with dilated ducts containing bile under pressure. Instill no more than 5 cc per pass if no duct is found.

9. If the initial pass is unsuccessful, reposition the needle successively in 10° increments caudally, then slightly more anteriorly or posteriorly (Fig. 1). To minimize damage to the liver capsule, the needle is not completely withdrawn from the liver prior to redirection.

10. Reinsertion may be repeated from 6 to 15 times before abandoning procedure. Most authors conclude that ducts are not dilated if no enlarged duct is found after six passes (3,5).

11. If the biliary tree is visualized, inject 15 to 60 cc of contrast to demonstrate the intrahepatic and extrahepatic bile ducts. Avoid overfilling of biliary system.
12. Take X-rays with fluoroscopy and overhead shots, including semierect shots for best visualization of the distal ducts. Normal ducts range from 3 to 7 mm for intrahepatic, 4 to 8 mm for common hepatic, and 5 to 11 mm for the common bile duct.
13. Aspirate at the end of the procedure. Decompression is particularly important with dilated ducts.
14. Send specimens for culture and cytologic study.

Interpretation (3)

Experience with PTC has shed light on specific fluoroscopic patterns that might affect interpretation of the procedure. When properly performed, PTC can allow visualization of 95% to 100% of dilated biliary ducts. Nondilated ducts are visualized in 60% to 95% of cases.

1. A linear tract of contrast is created on withdrawal of the needle during a pass. This may act as a conduit for preferential flow of contrast to venous structures that were already hit and divert contrast from smaller biliary radicles hit later.
2. The lymphatic pattern, serpiginous blood vessels, may be confused with sclerosing biliary radicles, although the course is different.
3. Some radicles may be adequate for filling the duct system and yet not be seen on fluoroscopy over the area of the common duct after each pass to look for filling.
4. Stagnant bile in the distal ducts can cause false proximal localization of the site of obstruction or may cause pseudodefects caused by poor admixture of contrast. This problem may be solved with delayed upright and/or prone films.
5. Dissection of dye through the adventitia of large vessels can be identified by slow flow in a broad pattern.

Postprocedure

1. Obtain a chest X-ray to rule out pneumothorax.
2. Monitor vital signs every hour × 6 hr then every 6 hr and

observe the patient for signs of hemorrhage, peritonitis, or sepsis.

3. Use antibiotics (see Preparation, Antibiotics) if there are dilated ducts with complete obstruction or if signs of sepsis or cholangitis develop.
4. A diagnosis of high-grade obstruction in conjunction with signs of complications usually requires internal (endoscopically placed) or external (percutaneously placed) biliary drainage. Rarely, emergent surgical drainage is required.

Complications (1–5,8–10)

Major complications are due to dilatation of ducts, not the number of passes (9). The incidence of complications increases if catheter drainage is performed (10).

Major

1. Fever and hypotension (2%).
2. Cholangitis with sepsis. Bacteremia most commonly occurs with gallstones, bile duct cancer, or pancreatic cancer.
3. Peritonitis (1–2%), with bile leakage in up to 5% in patients with obstruction.
4. Bleeding (1–2%). Forced respiration may increase the risk of bleeding due to capsular or parenchymal tear.
5. Bile embolism, with portal vein branch puncture (<1%).
6. Gallbladder puncture (<1%).

Minor (15% Incidence)

1. Subcapsular hematoma.
2. Capsular laceration.
3. Pneumothorax.
4. Transient but severe epigastric pain. This pain, caused by parenchymal extravasation, correlates with the number of passes. Local guarding may be found, and nausea and hypotension may develop, all clearing within 30 min with no sequelae.

REFERENCES

1. Hoevels J (1990): Percutaneous transhepatic cholangiography and percutaneous biliary drainage. In: *Interventional Radiology*, edited by R Dondelinger, et al, pp 187–199. Thieme Medical Publishers, New York.

2. Pereiras RJ, Chiprut R, Greenwald R, Schiff E (1977): Percutaneous transhepatic cholangiogaphy with the "skinny" needle. A rapid, simple, and accurate method in the diagnosis of cholestasis. *Ann Intern Med* 86:562–568.

3. Ferrucci JJ, Wittenberg J, Sarno R, Dreyfuss J (1976): Fine needle transhepatic cholangiography: a new approach to obstructive jaundice. *Am J Radiol* 127:403–407.

4. Harbin W, Mueller P, Ferrucci J (1980): Transhepatic cholangiography: complications and use patterns of the fine needle technique. *Radiology* 135:15–22.

5. Okuda K, Tanikawa K, Emura T, et al (1974): Nonsurgical, percutaneous transhepatic cholangiography: diagnostic significance in medical problems of the liver. *Am J Dig Dis* 19:21–36.

6. Barth K, Matsumoto A (1991): Patient care in interventional radiology: a perspective. *Radiology* 178:11–17.

7. Spies J, Rosen R, Lebowitz A (1988): Antibiotic prophylaxis in vascular and interventional radiology: a rational approach. *Radiology* 166: 381–387.

8. Cope C, Burke D, Meranze S (1990): *Atlas of Interventional Radiology*, pp 13.1–13.40. JB Lippincott Company, Philadelphia.

9. Jaques P, Mauro M, Scatliff J (1980): The failed transhepatic cholangiogram. *Radiology* 134:33–35.

10. Voegeli D, Crummy A, Weese J (1985): Percutaneous transhepatic cholangiography, drainage and biopsy in patients with malignant biliary obstruction. *Am J Surg* 150:243–247.

17 / Medications in the Gastrointestinal Procedure Unit

Kim L. Isaacs

Four classes of drugs are commonly used in the gastrointestinal (GI) procedures unit. These include:

1. Medications used to allay anxiety and discomfort: conscious sedation.
2. Local anesthetics to ease endoscopic passage.
3. Motility agents used to increase or decrease gastric motor function.
4. Antibiotics for subacute bacterial endocarditis (SBE) prophylaxis or to prevent postprocedure infection.

We will address each of these classes and discuss the use of some specific drugs.

Conscious Sedation

Recommendations

1. Meperidine, 25 to 50 mg intravenously (i.v.) initially with increments of 10 to 25 mg, and/or
2. Midazolam, 0.25 to 0.5 mg i.v. initially with increments of 0.25 to 0.5 mg.

Medications are used prior to and during certain endoscopic procedures to minimize patient anxiety and discomfort (1,2). The need for medication and the amount of medication are in part related to the patient's cultural background and past experiences. Age, underlying illness, and anticipated length of procedure also affect the amount of medication required for sedation. GI procedures in which conscious sedation is employed include upper GI endoscopic procedures, colonoscopy, endoscopic retrograde cholangiopancreatography (ERCP), percutaneous transhepatic cholangiograpy (PTC), and laparoscopy. Flexible sigmoidoscopy, motility studies, gastric secretory studies, and liver biopsy do not typically require periprocedure sedation.

Features of drugs used for conscious sedation include anxiolytic action, antegrade amnesia, quick onset of action, minimal effects on respiratory and cardiovascular systems, no venous irritation, and rapid recovery from its effects (1). Benzodiazepines offer many of these characteristics. Diazepam has been used extensively in endoscopic sedation. Midazolam is largely replacing diazepam due to its rapid elimination and water solubility leading to less venous irritation. Narcotics may be combined with midazolam. The effect of combination of narcotics and anxiolytics is more than additive, and adequate monitoring of respiratory and cardiovascular status is mandatory (3). Many institutions use a benzodiazapine alone for sedation. Our GI procedure unit uses a combination of meperidine and midazolam. In patients who are frail or elderly, meperidine alone is used due to the availability of a narcotic antagonist (naloxone), although with the availability of a benzodiazepine antagonist (flumazenil), benzodiazepines may receive increased usage. The goal of sedation is a relaxed, cooperative patient, not an unconscious one (2). With all sedated procedures, oxygen saturation is monitored with a pulse oximeter. Blood pressure and pulse are monitored throughout the procedure and documented. In patients who are at increased risk for cardiovascular and respiratory complications (i.e., cardiovascular disease, emphysema, preexisting arrhythmias) EKG tracing is also monitored (3,4).

Local Anesthetics

Recommendations

1. 1% Viscous lidocaine (Xylocaine), or
2. 20% Benzocaine spray, liquid, or gel (Hurricaine).

Topical anesthesia is used in upper endoscopic procedures to minimize discomfort in the posterior pharynx during endoscope passage. It also may help to decrease the gag response to posterior pharyngeal irritation. Topical anesthetics commonly used are a 20% benzocaine aerosolized solution and 1% viscous lidocaine. The onset of action occurs 15 to 30 sec after application so the anesthetic should be used immediately prior to passage of the endoscope to ensure effectiveness. Topical anesthesia is contraindicated in patients who have a known hypersensitivity to these agents.

Agents That Affect GI Motility

Recommendations

To decrease gastrointestinal motility: glucagon, 0.2 mg i.v. initially followed by 0.1- to 0.2-mg increments as needed.
To increase gastrointestinal motility: metoclopramide, single dose, i.v. given under 1 to 2 min.
  1. Adults: 10 mg i.v.
  2. Children (6–14): 2.5 to 5 mg i.v.
  3. Children under 6: 0.1 mg/kg i.v.

In certain situations (e.g., ERCP), it is helpful to decrease GI motility to improve visualization. Glucagon is used for this purpose. Glucagon is supplied as a powder and a 1.6% glycerin diluent and is mixed at a concentration of 1 mg/ml. Onset of action is approximately 1 min, with a duration of 9 to 17 min (5–7). Occasionally glucagon may induce nausea and vomiting (5).

To assist the passing of tubes (i.e., small intestinal biopsy capsules, feeding tubes) into the small intestine, the prokinetic agent, metoclopramide, may be used (8). If the tube has not passed the pylorus within 10 min using standard procedures, a *single dose* of metoclopramide is given i.v. over 1- to 2-min period. The onset of action is 1 to 3 min after an i.v. dose, with a duration of action of 1 to 2 hr (8). Diphenhydramine should be available to treat an acute dystonic reaction, although this would be uncommon using these small doses of metoclopramide.

Antibiotics

Antibiotics have several functions in the GI procedure unit. These include prophylaxis for SBE prophylaxis, prophylaxis for skin infection from surgical procedures, and prophylaxis to prevent ascending cholangitis during hepatobiliary procedures.

Subacute Bacterial Endocarditis Prophylaxis

Recommendations

Patients who need prophylaxis:

1. Patients with prosthetic valves.
2. Patients with prior bacterial endocarditis.
3. Patients with surgically created pulmonary/systemic shunts.
4. Patients with rheumatic or other valvular disease.
5. Patients with mitral valve prolapse who have valvular regurgitation.

Procedures that need prophylaxis:

1. Esophageal dilatation.
2. Variceal sclerosis.
3. Colonoscopy. (not recommended by the American Heart Association)
4. In other low-risk procedures such as esophagogastroduodenoscopy (EGD) with or without biopsy, prophylaxis may be used per physician discretion in high-risk patients (above).

Antibiotic Regimen (9)

Standard regimen:

1. Ampicillin, 2 g i.v. or intramuscularly (i.m.) and
2. Gentamicin, 1.5 mg/kg (do not exceed 80 mg) i.v. or i.m. 30 min before the procedure and
3. Amoxicillin, 1.5 g p.o., 6 hr after the initial dose or repeat the above parenteral regimen 8 hr after the original dose.

Penicillin allergic patients:

1. Vancomycin, 1 g given i.v. over 1 hr and
2. Gentamicin, 1.5 mg/kg (do not exceed 80 mg) i.v. or i.m. 1 hr before the procedure and may be repeated once 8 hr after the original dose.

Low-risk patient regimen:

1. Amoxicillin, 3 g orally 1 hr before the procedure followed by 1.5 g 6 hr after the initial dose.

Bacteremia has been well documented after diagnostic and therapeutic manipulation of the GI tract. It is estimated to occur in 4% of patients after upper GI endoscopy, compared to 82% with tooth extraction and 40% with brushing of teeth (10). Bacterial endocarditis is thought to occur following bacteremia in a patient who has a preexisting cardiac valvular lesion (9). The actual incidence of endocarditis following a GI procedure is very rare. There have been no controlled trials that address the efficacy of periprocedure antibiotic prophylaxis in preventing endocarditis. Taking these issues into consideration, the devastating effects of endocarditis make it reasonable to give prophylactic antibiotics to certain high-risk patients during procedures that have a high risk of transient bacteremia. The American Heart Association in 1990 published guidelines for prophylactic antibiotics in the prevention of bacterial endocarditis (9). Endoscopy with or without GI biopsy is included in the list of procedures not requiring SBE prophylaxis with the proviso that patients who have prosthetic heart valves, history of endocarditis, or surgically constructed systemic-pulmonary shunts may be given antibiotics as per physician discretion even in low-risk GI procedures. There is still some controversy in these recommendations. In general we follow the following guidelines as per the American Heart Association (9):

Surgical Prophylaxis (see Bozymski's chapter "Percutaneous Endoscopic Gastrostomy")

Recommendation

1. Cefazolin, 1 g i.v. 30 min before procedure. If the patient is already receiving antibiotics that cover skin pathogens, prophylactic treatment with cefazolin is not necessary.

The use of antibiotics for surgical wound prophylaxis has been studied extensively. The data show that there is a direct relationship between the efficacy of an antibiotic in preventing wound infection and the timing of its administration (11). In one study cefazolin administration significantly decreased the risk for wound infection after placement of a percutaneous endoscopic gastrostomy tube (12). Skin organisms such as *Staphylococcus aureus* are the most common contaminants of wounds in "clean" surgical procedures. Periostomal wound infection may occur in up to 30% of patients who undergo percutaneous endoscopic gastrostomy (12).

Biliary Tract Manipulation

General

The normal biliary tract does not contain bacteria whereas in up to one-half of abnormal biliary trees (strictures, stones), microorganisms can be cultured. The biliary system is most commonly colonized with gram-negative enteric bacteria (*Escherichia coli*, *Klebsiella*, *Enterobacter*) and less commonly, enterococcus, *Pseudomonas*, and *Clostridium* (13,14). Patients who have cholangitis or infection of the pancreatic or biliary tree should be on antibiotics to treat that infection regardless of the procedure being performed.

Percutaneous Transhepatic Cholangiography (see chapter by Isaacs and Levinson)

Recommendations (15,16)

1. Cefoperazone, 2 g i.v. 1 hr prior to procedure or
2. Mezlocillin, 3 g i.v. 1 hr prior to procedure or
3. Ampicillin, 2 g i.v., and gentamicin, 1.5 mg/kg i.v., 1 hr prior to procedure or
4. Cefoxitin, 1 g i.v. 1 hr prior to procedure (17).

Antibiotics are recommended prior to PTC. There are multiple regimens in the radiology literature that are recommended to cover common biliary organisms. Some authors recommend ceftriaxone (15,16) for outpatients due to its high serum levels for 24 hr; however, it should be recognized that ceftriaxone has been associated with increased incidence of biliary sludge.

Endoscopic Retrograde Cholangiopancreatography (see Bozymski's chapter "Endoscopic Retrograde Cholangiopancreatography")

Recommendations

1. See PTC recommendations or
2. Ampicillin/sulbactam (2 g/1 g) i.v. 1 to 2 hr preprocedure and 8 hr after the initial dose.

When Should Prophylaxis Be Given?

1. Sphincterotomy.
2. Stone extraction.
3. Placement of a biliary endoprosthesis.
4. Diagnosis study of an obstructed system (e.g., sclerosis cholangitis with strictures).

In patients who are undergoing diagnostic ERCP with no suspected infection or obstruction, specific preprocedure biliary prophylaxis is not required. Biliary antibiotic prophylaxis is recommended in all cases of biliary obstruction where manipulation of the bile duct is anticipated, including sphincterotomy, stone extraction, and placement of a biliary endoprosthesis. Prophylactic antibiotics are given 1 to 2 hr before the procedure and are continued for 12 hr after the procedure. There are multiple antibiotic regimens that may be used successfully for biliary prophylaxis. The regimens for PTC should be equally as effective for biliary tract prophylaxis in ERCP. Other regimens that have been used with some success include: (a) cefoxitin, 1 g i.v. (17) and (b) ampicillin/sulbactam (2 g/1 g) i.v. 1 to 2 hr before procedure and again 8 hr after the initial dose (13). The exact combination of antibiotics is not as critical as the timing of administration and the provision of adequate coverage for biliary organisms.

REFERENCES

1. Lauven P (1990): Pharmacology of drugs for conscious sedation. *Scand J Gastroenterol Suppl* 179:1–6.

2. McCloy R, Pearson R (1990): A review of benzodiazepine sedation and its reversal in endoscopy. *Scand J Gastroenterol Suppl* 179:7–11.
3. Fleischer D (1989): Monitoring the patient receiving conscious sedation for gastrointestinal endoscopy. Issues and guidelines. *Gastrointest Endosc* 35:262–266.
4. Bell G (1990): Monitoring—the gastroenterologist's view. *Scand J Gastroenterol Suppl* 179:18–23.
5. Chernish S, Maglinte D (1990): Glucagon: common untoward reactions—review and recommendations. *Radiology* 177:145–146.
6. Feczko P, Haggear A, Halpert R (1986): A reappraisal of upper gastrointestinal response to low-dose glucagon. *Crit Rev Diagn Imaging* 23:377–412.
7. Gerner T, Myren J, Larsen S (1983): Premedication in upper gastrointestinal endoscopy. *Scand J Gastroenterol* 18:925–928.
8. McCallum R (1985): Review of the current status of prokinetic agents in gastroenterology. *Am J Gastroenterol* 80:1008–1016.
9. Dajani A, Bisno A, Chung K, et al (1990): Prevention of bacterial endocarditis: recommendations by the American Heart Association. *JAMA* 264:2919–2922.
10. Mamel J (1990): Prophylactic antibiotics in GI endoscopy. *Contemp Gastroenterol* 3:37–40.
11. Kaiser A (1986): Antibiotic prophylaxis in surgery. *N Engl J Med* 315:1129–1138.
12. Jain N, Larson D, Shroeder K, et al (1987): Antibiotic prophylaxis for percutaneous endoscopic gastrostomy: a prospective, randomized, double-blind clinical trial. *Ann Intern Med* 107:824–828.
13. Edwards G, Lindsay G, Taylor E, Group WoSSISG (1990): A bacteriological assessment of ampicillin with sulbactam as antibiotic prophylaxis in patients undergoing biliary tract operations. *J Hosp Infect* 16:249–255.
14. Levine J, Botet J, Kurtz R (1990): Microbiological analysis of sepsis complicating non-surgical biliary drainage in malignant obstruction. *Gastrointest Endosc* 36:364–368.
15. Barth K, Matsumoto A (1991): Patient care in interventional radiology: a perspective. *Radiology* 178:11–17.
16. Spies J, Rosen R, Lebowitz A (1988): Antibiotic prophylaxis in vascular and interventional radiology: a rational approach. *Radiology* 166:381–387.
17. Maki D, Lammers J, Aughey D (1984): Comparative studies of multiple-dose cefoxitin vs. single-dose cefonicid for surgical prophylaxis in patients undergoing biliary tract operations or hysterectomy. *Rev Infect Dis* 6 (suppl 4):S887.

18 / Upper Gastrointestinal Endoscopy

R. Balfour Sartor

Upper gastrointestinal (GI) endoscopy has revolutionized clinical gastroenterology by providing a rapid means of accurate diagnosis, and has vast potential for research and therapeutic applications. The purpose of this chapter is to provide an overview of upper GI endoscopy. It is not intended to be a comprehensive source of instruction. Endoscopic technique and interpretation are best taught by an experienced endoscopist, supplemented by a review of recent inclusive texts (1–3) that outline technique and pathology in detail.

Indications

The indications for upper GI endoscopy are too numerous to outline completely and must be individualized (4–6). The major indications follow.

Diagnostic

1. To establish the site of upper GI bleeding.
2. To visually define and biopsy abnormalities seen on upper GI series (ulcers, filling defects, and cancers).
3. To evaluate healing of treated gastric ulcers.
4. To evaluate dysphagia, dyspepsia, abdominal pain, gastric outlet obstruction; chest pain after negative cardiac evaluation; and iron deficiency anemia after negative colonoscopy.
5. To evaluate odynophagia in immunosuppressed states.
6. To determine extent of damage after caustic ingestion.

131

Therapeutic

1. Gastric, duodenal, and esophageal polypectomy.
2. Removal of foreign bodies.
3. Disintegration of bezoars.
4. Treatment of bleeding ulcers with electrocautery, heat probes, laser, or injection therapy.
5. Sclerotherapy of esophageal varices.
6. Placement of guide wires or balloons for esophageal and gastric dilatation.
7. Placement of small intestinal feeding tubes and percutaneous gastrostomy catheters.

Contraindications

Absolute

1. Shock (unless preoperative to guide emergent surgical therapy).
2. Acute myocardial infarction.
3. Severe dyspnea with hypoxemia.
4. Coma (unless patient is intubated).
5. Seizures.
6. Acutely perforated ulcer or perforated esophagus.
7. Atlantoaxial subluxation.

Relative

1. Uncooperative patient.
2. Coagulopathy:
   a. Prothrombin time 3 sec over control.
   b. Partial thromboplastin time (PTT) 20 sec over control.
   c. Bleeding time >10 min.
   d. Platelet count <100,000/mm^3.
3. Zenker's diverticulum.
4. Upper esophageal stricture.
5. Myocardial ischemia.
6. Thoracic aortic aneurysm.

Preparation

1. The patient should have nothing by mouth for 6 to 8 hr prior to the procedure.
2. Review the patient's chart, including X-rays and coagulation studies.
3. See the patient prior to the procedure. Be certain the study is indicated and that the patient understands the risks and benefits and agrees to the procedure.
4. Write a preprocedure note.
5. Obtain written, informed consent; start the intravenous (i.v.) line; anesthetize the patient's throat with a topical agent; and attach the pulse oximeter.
6. Administer meperidine, up to 50 mg i.v., slowly.
7. If needed, administer midazolam (0.75–2 mg) or diazepam (2–10 mg) i.v. slowly until an appropriate level of sedation is reached. Since the effects of meperidine can be rapidly reversed with naloxone, we prefer this drug to midazolam or diazepam. Diazepam also has a high incidence of phlebitis, especially when infused into a small vein of the hand. Watch the patient carefully for respiratory depression and give preoperative medication cautiously in elderly and malnourished patients. Many patients undergoing diagnostic endoscopy with small-caliber scopes need little if any sedation.

Equipment

1. Endoscope of choice. We use a small-caliber endoscope routinely and reserve use of the larger endoscopes for anticipated biopsies or therapeutic procedures.
2. Light source.
3. Teaching head (or monitor for video endoscopy).
4. Biopsy forceps.
5. Cytology brush.
6. Washing cannula and syringe.
7. Camera (or disc for video endoscopy).

Procedure

Passing the Endoscope

1. Administer medication so that patient is sedated but alert enough to assist in swallowing.
2. Place the recumbent patient in the left lateral position with bite block in place.
3. Hold the scope with the left hand on the controls and the right hand on the shaft at the 25- to 30-cm mark in a partially flexed (60°) configuration.
4. With the patient's neck partially flexed, pass the endoscope through the hypopharynx. Under direct visualization using light pressure, slowly guide the tip of the scope past the epiglottis to rest on the cricopharyngeus, which is located in the midline posterior to the larynx and between the pyriform sinuses, 15 to 18 cm from the incisors (Fig. 1). Gently insert the endoscope into the esophageal lumen during relaxation of the cricopharyngeus as the patient swallows. Be certain to keep the scope in the midline, out of the pyriform sinuses, and posterior to the larynx.
5. Once the scope has passed the upper esophageal sphincter (20 cm), advance it under *direct vision* at all times and with only enough air insufflation to permit visualization.

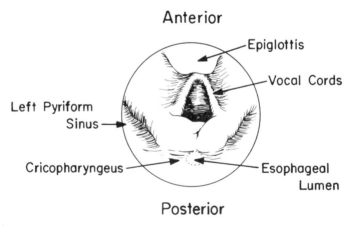

Anterior

Epiglottis

Vocal Cords

Left Pyriform Sinus →

Cricopharyngeus →

← Esophageal Lumen

Posterior

FIG. 1. View of the hypopharynx and laryngeal structures during endoscopic intubation. The cricopharyngeus is posterior at the 6 o'clock position.

Visualization of Esophagus, Stomach, and Duodenum

1. Advance the scope through the distal esophagus, identifying the gastroesophageal junction by the change from white to coral-colored mucosa ("Z" line) and the lower esophageal sphincter. The level of the diaphragm can be determined by asking the patient to sniff. A hiatal hernia is present if the gastroesophageal junction and gastric folds are significantly above the level of the diaphragm. Barrett's esophagus is identified by an irregular Z line with fingers or islands of red gastric epithelium extending into the tan-colored esophageal mucosa.

2. Observe the motility of the stomach, particularly the antrum, for asymmetry and fixation, as subtle invasive lesions are sometimes suspected from damping of gastric contractions.

3. Insert the scope through the pyloric channel into the duodenal bulb, then into the second portion of the duodenum by torquing and turning the tip posteriorly (to the right).

4. The duodenal bulb and pyloric channel are visualized best by slowly withdrawing the scope while rotating the tip by torquing the shaft from side to side. Pay particular attention to the superior and posterior portions of the duodenal bulb.

5. Returning to the stomach, pay special attention to the angulus and the gastroesophageal junction, visualizing both by retroflexion as well as by forward viewing. The endoscope is retroflexed by maximally turning the tip upward so that it is in a J shape. By rotating the retroflexed scope, the entire gastric cardia can be thoroughly visualized.

6. After thoroughly evaluating the stomach by slowly withdrawing the scope while rotating the tip in a 360° fashion, remove the excess air from the stomach by suction to minimize abdominal distension.

Biopsy

1. To obtain adequate depth of sampling, gently compress the open biopsy forceps against the mucosa.

2. It is not necessary to biopsy a routine duodenal bulbar ulcer unless lymphoma is suspected or nodularity or a mass is seen.

3. A gastric ulcer always should be biopsied, unless it is a channel ulcer or prepyloric erosion that is clearly benign. Biopsy the *margin* of the ulcer in all four quadrants, the base several times, and the mucosa next to the ulcer (i.e., at least six to eight biopsies) as demonstrated in Figure 2. Do not biopsy if the patient has evidence of active or recent bleeding from the ulcer (clot on the base or visible vessel).

4. Do not biopsy the esophageal mucosa if the patient is to have an esophageal dilatation within a week of the endoscopy. Use the brush for cytology only. However, biopsies can be safely performed *after* dilatation.

5. Biopsies of the distal esophagus should be performed at least 2 cm above the gastroesophageal junction to minimize the mistaken diagnosis of Barrett's (columnar) epithelium or esophagitis. Esophageal biopsies can be obtained more easily by turning the tip of the scope toward the mucosa.

6. If the biopsy forceps does not pass through the distal channel, straighten the endoscope and try again.

7. Larger biopsies of polypoid lesions can be obtained with a snare cautery or "hot" biopsy technique.

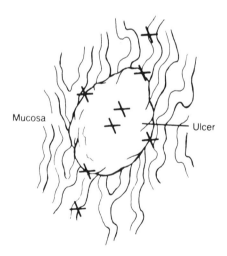

FIG. 2. Sites for biopsying a gastric ulcer. Biopsies (×) should be taken from each of the four quadrants of the margin, the base, and the surrounding gastric mucosa.

Cytology

Cytologic examination of possible malignant lesions will complement biopsies by increasing their yield of positive results.

1. Obtain cytologic specimens before biopsies to diminish dilution of cells by blood. Brush suspicious areas (gastric ulcers, mucosal masses) to obtain adequate cellular material. The use of a disposable, retractable brush protected by a plastic sheath will protect the sample from being lost in the biopsy channel of the endoscope.
2. Stroke the brush over a Dakin slide moistened with normal saline.
3. Place the slide in preservative in a Pap smear bottle.
4. Submucosal cytologic specimens can be obtained from mass lesions by aspiration of saline through a sclerotherapy needle inserted into the lesion.
5. Lesions to be brushed should be cleansed of surface mucus, blood, and exudate by a jet of water through the biopsy channel.

Subacute Bacterial Endocarditis Prophylaxis

Prophylaxis is probably indicated for prosthetic heart valves but not for damaged natural valves in patients undergoing diagnostic endoscopy. Because biopsies and sclerotherapy increase the risk of bacteremia, patients with damaged heart valves who undergo therapeutic endoscopy or biopsies should receive prophylactic antibiotics. See the chapter by Isaacs, "Medications in the Gastrointestinal Procedure Unit," for antibiotic protocols.

Miscellaneous

1. In patients with achalasia, the esophagus should be emptied of retained food prior to endoscopy via a large-diameter tube and lavage. This will permit better visualization and prevent aspiration.
2. If esophageal varices are encountered and are not clinically suspected, make sure they are *carefully* documented by multiple observers and photographs.

3. Rapidly developed photographs should be attached to the procedure note to allow the referring physician to visualize the morphologic findings.
4. Antral biopsies for *Helicobacter pylori* should be considered in patients with refractory or complicated peptic ulcer disease or persistent gastritis.

Postprocedure

1. Fill out a procedure sheet and write a summary note in the medical record.
2. Give nothing by mouth until the gag reflex and sensation in the throat return.
3. The patient should not drive for 6 to 8 hr after conscious sedation. Detailed instructions should be given since many patients do not recall verbal discussions after sedation.

Complications

Overall complication rates of the procedure and the medications are in the range of 0.1% to 0.2%, with mortality in the range of 0.014% to 0.065% (7,8).

1. Drug-induced:
   a. Respiratory arrest (0.07%).
   b. Phlebitis.
2. Perforation (0.033%–0.1%). The most common sites are the pharynx, upper esophagus, and stomach.
3. Bleeding (0.03%). This is from biopsies, dislodging clots from bleeding points, and Mallory-Weiss tears induced by retching during endoscopy.
4. Aspiration (0.08%). The risk can be decreased by giving the patient nothing by mouth, lavaging patients with bleeding or achalasia, and using minimum air insufflation.
5. Retropharyngeal hematomas and crush injuries.
6. Infection:
   a. Transient bacteremia (5%). There is only one case report of endocarditis induced by endoscopy.
   b. There is no evidence of hepatitis B or acquired immu-

nodeficiency syndrome (AIDS) being transmitted by properly cleaned scopes (9).

7. Complications to the endoscopist:
   a. Bitten finger.
   b. Herpetic conjunctivitis.
   c. Because of the potential transmission of hepatitis and AIDS viruses, we suggest that gloves, gown, and mask be worn at all times and that all specimens be handled in accordance with universal precaution guidelines.

REFERENCES

1. Sivak MV (1987): *Gastroenterologic Endoscopy.* WB Saunders Company, Philadelphia.
2. Silverstein FE, Tytgat GNJ (1987): *Atlas of Gastrointestinal Endoscopy.* WB Saunders Company, Philadelphia.
3. Blackstone MO (1984): *Endoscopic Interpretation.* Raven Press, New York.
4. American Society for Gastrointestinal Endoscopy (1989): *Appropriate Use of Gastrointestinal Endoscopy.* Manchester, Massachusetts.
5. Morrissey JF, Reichelderfer M (1991): Gastrointestinal endoscopy. *N Engl J Med* 325:1142–1149.
6. Tytgat G (1991): Upper gastrointestinal endoscopy. In: *Textbook of Gastroenterology,* edited by T Yamada, DH Alpers, C Owyang, DN Powell, FE Silverstein, pp 2225–2247. JB Lippincott Company, Philadelphia.
7. Shamir M, Schuman BM (1980): Complications of fiberoptic endoscopy. *Gastrointest Endosc* 26:86–91.
8. Arrowsmith JB, Gerstman BB, Fleischer DE, Benjamin SB (1991): Results from the American Society for Gastrointestinal Endoscopy/U.S. Food and Drug Administration collaborative study on complication rates and drug use during gastrointestinal endoscopy. *Gastrointest Endosc* 37:421–427.
9. Villa E, Pasquinelli C, Rigo G, et al (1984): Gastrointestinal endoscopy and HBV infection: no evidence for a causal relationship. *Gastrointest Endosc* 30:15–17.

19 / Emergency Upper Gastrointestinal Endoscopy

R. Balfour Sartor

Early esophagogastroduodenoscopy can determine the source of bleeding in upper gastrointestinal (GI) hemorrhage approximately 90% of the time (1–3). It is particularly useful in detecting mucosal lesions that cannot be seen by barium contrast radiography, such as Mallory-Weiss tears, gastritis, and esophagitis. However, routine diagnostic endoscopy has not been demonstrated to improve the mortality or morbidity associated with routine upper GI hemorrhage that ceases spontaneously in 85% to 95% of cases (4,5), although it may be helpful in continued or recurrent bleeding (1–3). Therefore, emergency endoscopy should be performed only when it will influence a clinical decision such as medical or surgical therapy or when endoscopic hemostasis is required. Otherwise, the procedure can be performed electively with greater safety and improved visualization. For detailed information on therapeutic endoscopic intervention for bleeding ulcers or varices, see the chapters by Drossman, "Ablation of Bleeding (Nonvariceal) Gastrointestinal Lesions," and by Bozymski, "Endoscopic Sclerosis of Esophageal Varices," and two publications (6,7).

Indications

1. Active upper GI bleeding (recent hematemesis or blood aspirated from the stomach with nasogastric suction).
2. Massive rectal bleeding in which a duodenal ulcer is strongly suspected.
3. The patient with an abdominal aortic graft who has bled, to diagnose a possible aortoenteric fistula.

Contraindications

(See the chapter by Sartor, "Upper Gastrointestinal Endoscopy," Contraindications.) To prevent complications, stabilize the patient hemodynamically prior to the procedure. Be particularly attentive for:

1. EKG evidence of ischemia.
2. Hypovolemia.
3. Inability to cooperate.
4. Severe anemia.

Preparation

1. Decide if the patient is stable enough for endoscopy.
2. Correct severe hypovolemia or anemia with blood transfusions and intravenous (i.v.) fluids.
3. Lavage with large volumes of saline or water using a large tube (Ewald) to remove as many clots as possible. The standard Levine nasogastric tube is inadequate for clot removal. If during the lavage there is no return, do not forcibly aspirate; put in more saline. The gastric mucosa can be traumatized easily by overly aggressive aspiration.
4. Obtain consent for endoscopy and possible therapeutic procedures (esophageal sclerotherapy or coagulation of bleeding site) from the patient or a close relative.
5. Anesthetize the pharynx with a topical agent.
6. Administer premedication (see the chapter by Isaacs, "Medications in the Gastrointestinal Procedure Unit") with greater caution in patients with decreased cardiorespiratory reserve or altered mental status.

Equipment

1. Portable cart for transporting equipment.
2. Endoscope—use an endoscope with a large suction channel to facilitate clot removal and washing. A double channelled endoscope is optimal for therapeutic procedures.
3. Light source.
4. Teaching head or portable video monitor.

5. Camera or video disc.
6. Washing cannula and syringe.
7. Sclerotherapy (see Bozymski's chapter "Endoscopic Sclerosis of Esophageal Varices") and coagulation equipment.
8. Pulse oximeter and cardiac monitor.

Procedure

1. If possible, arrange for the procedure to be done in the emergency room or intensive care unit, where there is adequate support for the unstable patient.
2. Pass the endoscope under direct vision as for an elective endoscopy (see Procedure in chapter by Sartor, "Upper Gastrointestinal Endoscopy").
3. Have a nurse or assistant available at all times during the procedure to observe the patient's vital signs and to suction secretions and regurgitated material.
4. After introduction of the scope, inspect the distal esophagus; then go straight to the duodenum, scanning the lesser curvature of the gastric mucosa as you go. The three most important findings are esophageal varices, diffuse gastritis, and duodenal ulcer [treatment is different (sclerotherapy) for varices; surgery should be deferred in diffuse gastritis; surgery or endoscopic intervention is indicated earlier in peptic ulcer disease]. Then, if the patient becomes uncooperative, the most important areas will have been seen.
5. Be certain to visualize the gastric cardia by retroflexing the scope to identify Mallory-Weiss tears and gastric varices.
6. A large pool of clots will usually obscure the greater curvature of the fundus. The patient can be rotated on his or her back or right side to visualize this area better, but extensive pre-endoscopic lavage is well worth the time.
7. Emergency upper endoscopy is not successful in demonstrating the bleeding lesion in 5% to 10% of cases, owing to either clots or active bleeding obscuring the bleeding site or patient noncompliance. In these cases, it is not productive to prolong the procedure and risk aspiration or other complications. It is very helpful to know the approximate location of bleeding and whether diffuse gastritis or varices are present, even if the exact bleeding point is not demonstrated.

8. If there is active bleeding, call a surgeon before endoscopy to see the lesion in order to facilitate early surgery. Treatment of the bleeding lesion with a heat probe, electrocoagulator, laser, submucosal epinephrine injection, or sclerotherapy may be indicated.
9. A nasogastric tube and gastric lavage will almost always induce areas of trauma in the fundus. Be cautious of calling erythematous areas gastric erosions when there is no exudate to indicate chronic inflammation.
10. If an ulcer is identified, look for stigmata of recent hemorrhage that indicate a high risk of continued or recurrent bleeding. These stigmata include a protruding visible vessel, an adherent clot, a black eschar, or actual bleeding (9).
11. Exert caution to prevent exposure to potential infectious blood by wearing gloves, gown, mask, and eye protection.

Postprocedure

1. Suction water through the endoscope immediately after the procedure to prevent blockage of the suction channel with clots.
2. Retrieve and clean all equipment.
3. Fill out a procedure sheet and write a summary note in the medical record.

Complications

The risk of major complications in emergency endoscopy is 0.59% (10), which is three to six times the risk during elective procedures.

Perforation (0.26%)

Usually involves ulcers.

Aspiration (0.2%)

This is higher than in elective endoscopy because the stomach is full of clots, and the patient's sensorium is frequently diminished.

Hemorrhage (0.13%)

Usually occurs with varices or during attempts to expose a vessel in an ulcer crater.

REFERENCES

1. Gilbert DA, Silverstein FE (1987): Endoscopy in gastrointestinal bleeding. In: *Gastroenterologic Endoscopy*, edited by MV Sivak, Jr, pp 110–127. WB Saunders Company, Philadelphia.
2. Morrissey JF, Reichelderfer M (1991): Gastrointestinal endoscopy. *N Engl J Med* 325:1142–1149.
3. Tytgat G (1991): Upper gastrointestinal endoscopy. In: *Textbook of Gastroenterology*, edited by T Yamada, DH Alpers, C Owyang, DN Powell, FE Silverstein, pp 2225–2247. JB Lippincott Company, Philadelphia.
4. Peterson WL, Barnett CC, Smith HJ, Allen MH, Corbett DB (1981): Routine upper endoscopy in upper gastrointestinal bleeding: a randomized controlled trial. *N Engl J Med* 304:925–929.
5. Graham DY (1980): Limited value of early endoscopy in the management of acute upper gastrointestinal bleeding: prospective controlled trial. *Am J Surg* 140:284–290.
6. Sikas SE, ed (1990): *Therapeutic Gastrointestinal Endoscopy*. Igaku-Shoin, New York.
7. Berkin JS, O'Phelan CA, eds (1990): *Advanced Therapeutic Endoscopy*. Raven Press, New York.
8. Consensus Development Panel (1990): Consensus statement on therapeutic endoscopy and bleeding ulcers. *Gastrointest Endosc* 36:S62–S65.
9. Storey DW, Brown SE, Swain CP, et al (1981): Endoscopic prediction of recurrent bleeding in peptic ulcers. *N Engl J Med* 305:915–916.
10. Gilbert DA, Silverstein FE, Tedesco FJ (1981): National ASGE Survey on upper gastrointestinal bleeding: complications of endoscopy. *Dig Dis Sci* 26(Suppl):55–59S.

20 / Mucosal Biopsy of the Duodenum and Small Bowel in Adult Patients and Duodenal Aspiration

William D. Heizer

In most centers, endoscopic biopsy at the distal second duodenum has replaced suction biopsy at the ligament of Treitz for the diagnosis of small-bowel mucosal disease (1–6). Although the endoscopic biopsy specimens are not as large as those obtained with the suction instrument, diagnostic accuracy is reported to be comparable if at least four specimens are obtained through the endoscope using forceps of adequate size (at least 8 mm across the open jaws). Advantages of the endoscopic method over suction biopsy techniques include: (a) certainty of obtaining tissue, (b) absence of radiation exposure for patient and staff, (c) less time-consuming, and (d) expertise is more widely available. Disadvantages of the endoscopic approach include: (a) generally done under conscious sedation which increases risk, (b) small mucosal specimens that are difficult to orient and have crush artifact, and (c) higher charge except where there is a different (lower) charge for endoscopic biopsy than for diagnostic endoscopy (4). The change from suction to endoscopic biopsy is likely to increase the new case detection rate for celiac sprue and probably for other mucosal abnormalities but at the expense of a fall in the percentage of biopsy specimens obtained that are abnormal (6). If a suction biopsy is desired, the Carey capsule technique described for pediatric patients (see Ulshen's chapter, "Small-Bowel Biopsy in Pediatric Patients") should be used. The multipurpose tube (Rubin-Quinton) is no longer being manufactured.

Indications

Small-Bowel Biopsy

Indicated when it is important to support, confirm, or exclude diseases of the small intestine (7,8). Diagnostic biopsies may be appropriate not only for the classic symptoms of malabsorption (diarrhea and weight loss) but also for other signs and symptoms of gluten-sensitive enteropathy (anemia, osteopenia, bone pain) and Whipple's disease (arthritis, serositis, and central nervous system dysfunction). Mucosal biopsies are also indicated when endoscopic findings suggestive of gluten-sensitive enteropathy are incidentally found. These include a reduced number of folds of Kerckring in the second duodenum (9), loss of the velvety appearance on close-up view of the mucosa (10), and "coarse or notched" appearance of the folds of Kerckring (11).

Duodenal Aspiration

1. To diagnose bacterial overgrowth.
2. To determine the presence of cholesterol crystals or white blood cells in patients with suspected gallbladder disease.
3. To diagnose giardiasis. However, if a duodenal biopsy specimen is obtained, a touch prep or smear of the specimen on a glass slide is an equally good or better way to make this diagnosis. If endoscopy is not needed, an appropriate way to obtain a sample of duodenal fluid to test for giardiasis is with a string test (Entero-test, HDC Corporation, 2551 Casey Avenue, Mountain View, California 94043).

Contraindications

1. Uncooperative patient.
2. Uncorrectable coagulation disorder.

Preparation

1. Same as for upper endoscopy (see Sartor's chapter, "Upper Gastrointestinal Endoscopy").

Equipment

1. Upper endoscope with a biopsy channel at least 2.35 mm in diameter and preferably 2.8 or 3.7 mm in diameter.
2. Biopsy forceps suitable for the endoscope. The open jaws of the biopsy forceps should be 8 or 9 mm across.
3. Monofilament, high-density, polyethylene mesh from: National Filter Media Corporation, P.O. Box 156, 969 North Third Street, West Salt Lake City, Utah 84110; Catalog No. 20402899 (32 × 32 filaments/in.) or Catalog No. 2040299 (52 × 52 filaments/in.).
4. Paraformaldehyde or other suitable fixative.

Procedure

1. Using the papilla of Vater as a landmark, take at least four biopsy specimens, approximately 1 cm apart, distal to the papilla in the second or third duodenum.
2. Take biopsy specimens from the crest of the folds of Kerckring in order to fill the biopsy cup and obtain the largest specimen possible.
3. If the sample size is not adequate, try the "turn and suction" technique described by Levine and Reid (12) or the "push-off" technique described by Gowen (13). However, usually it is best just to obtain a larger number of specimens, even up to 8 or 10, or to use an endoscope with a 3.7-mm-diameter channel that will accommodate a larger forceps.
4. Opinion is mixed about how much effort, if any, should be made to orient the specimens. One approach is to take a large number of specimens, minimum of four, in order to increase the chance that at least one will be adequately oriented. The other approach is to use a needle or small forceps to pry open the specimen, which is usually curled into a ball with the villous surface on the outside. Using a gloved finger or other suitable surface, flatten out the specimen, mucosa side down. Gently transfer the specimen to the monofilament mesh, with the cut surface touching the mesh, and place it in the fixative (see also Ulshen's chapter, "Small-Bowel Biopsy in Pediatric Patients"). An inexperienced person can severely dam-

age the mucosal surface when using this technique. We make only a brief and gentle attempt to orient the specimen before putting it on the monofilament mesh and in the fixative.

Postprocedure

Same as for upper endoscopy.

Complications

Same as for upper endoscopy. The risk of bleeding is probably increased by multiple biopsies. However, we are not aware of any reported instances of bleeding secondary to endoscopic biopsies of duodenal mucosa.

Duodenal Aspiration

1. To obtain fluid for quantitative culture for bacterial overgrowth, endoscopically cannulate the duodenum and pass a clean catheter through the biopsy channel.
2. Aspirate fluid through the catheter directly into a sterile syringe.
3. Push air out of the syringe and take it to the lab for quantitative anaerobic and aerobic culture of the fluid.
4. If there is no fluid present, reposition the patient with the right side down. Nevertheless, patients may not have enough fluid in the duodenum to aspirate, especially those who do not have a motor disorder of the upper intestine.
5. To obtain bile, place the tip of the endoscope near the papilla of Vater. If necessary, inject cholecystokinin (0.02 μg/kg) subcutaneously or instill 35 cc of 35% magnesium sulfate solution into the distal portion of the second duodenum through the endoscope to stimulate gallbladder emptying.

REFERENCES

1. Holdstock G, Eade OE, Isaacson P, Smith CL (1979): Endoscopic duodenal biopsies in coeliac disease and duodenitis. *Scand J Gastroenterol* 14:717–720.

2. Scott BB, Jenkins D (1981): Endoscopic small intestinal biopsy. *Gastrointest Endosc* 27:162–167.
3. Mee AS, Burke M, Vallon AG, Newman J, Cotton PB (1985): Small bowel biopsy for malabsorption: comparison of the diagnostic adequacy of endoscopic forceps and capsule biopsy specimens. *Br Med J* 291: 679–772.
4. Achkar E, Carey WD, Petras R, Sivak MV (1986): Comparison of suction capsules and endoscopic biopsy of small bowel mucosa. *Gastrointest Endosc* 32:278–281.
5. Smith JA, Mayberry JF, Ansell ID, Long RG (1989): Small bowel biopsy for disaccharidase levels: evidence that endoscopic forceps biopsy can replace the Crosby capsule. *Clin Chim Acta* 183:317–322.
6. Saverymuttu SH, Sabbat J, Burke M, Maxwell JD (1991): Impact of endoscopic duodenal biopsy on the detection of small intestinal villous atrophy. *Postgrad Med J* 67:47–49.
7. Rubin CE, Dobbins WO (1965): Per oral biopsy of the small intestine. A review of its diagnostic usefulness. *Gastroenterology* 49:676–697.
8. Perea DR, Weinstein WM, Rubin CE (1975): Small intestinal biopsy. *Hum Pathol* 6:157–217.
9. Broochi E, Corazza GR, Caletti G, Treggiari EA, Barbara L, Gasbarrini G (1986): Endoscopic demonstration of loss of duodenal folds in the diagnosis of celiac disease. *N Engl J Med* 319:741–744.
10. Stevens FM, McCarthy CF (1976): The endoscopic demonstration of coeliac disease. *Endoscopy* 8:177–180.
11. Sanflippo G, Patane R, Fusto A, Passanisi G, Valenti R, Russo A (1986): Endoscopic approach to childhood coeliac disease. *Acta Gastroenterol Belg* 49:401–408.
12. Levine DS, Reid BJ (1991): Endoscopic biopsy technique for acquiring larger mucosal samples. *Gastrointest Endosc* 37:332–337.
13. Gowen GF (1986): An improved technique of endoscopic biopsy in the upper gastrointestinal tract. *Gastrointest Endosc* 32:59–60.

21 / Endoscopic Retrograde Cholangiopancreatography

Eugene M. Bozymski

Endoscopic retrograde cholangiopancreatography (ERCP) is a standard procedure used in the diagnosis and treatment of certain diseases of the biliary tree and pancreas. Along with outlining the common bile duct, the intrahepatic ducts, and the gallbladder, one can also visualize the pancreatic ductal system. In addition to a skilled endoscopist, a radiologist with special interest in this area is very helpful in obtaining the maximum information from this procedure.

In cases of obstructive jaundice, the merits of percutaneous transhepatic cholangiography versus ERCP should be debated with respect to the individual patient, keeping in mind the expertise and limitations of the available professional staff. However, there are very few instances in which a gastroenterologist capable of performing ERCP is not readily available and this nearly always is the indicated procedure. Generally, diagnostic ERCP should be done only by those capable of proceeding with indicated endoscopic therapeutic interventions.

Indications

1. Evaluation of the patient with suspected obstructive jaundice.
2. Evaluation for suspected disease of the intrahepatic or extrahepatic biliary system.
3. Evaluation of the patient with suspected pancreatic cancer.
4. Evaluation of recurrent pancreatitis of unknown etiology.
5. To determine the anatomy of the pancreas and its ductal system prior to operative, radiologic, or endoscopic intervention

for chronic pancreatitis, suspected pancreatic trauma, or pseudocyst or other pancreaticobiliary disorders.

Contraindications

1. Significant bleeding diathesis.
2. Recent acute pancreatitis, unless surgery or endoscopic sphincterotomy is planned for suspected choledocholithiasis.

Preparation

1. Surgical consultation generally is appropriate.
2. Make certain that there is no barium in the gastrointestinal tract [computed tomography (CT) scan, barium enema] that will obscure the field.
3. Obtain an informed, written consent.
4. Place an intravenous (i.v.) line in the right arm with the port close to the vein for administration of atropine, meperidine, midazolam, and glucagon.
5. Have the patient lie on the left side with the left arm behind the back to facilitate the roll to the prone position.
6. Place the patient on preprocedure systemic antibiotics if cholangitis or infection in the pancreatic or biliary tree is suspected. Antibiotic combinations for sepsis frequently used include tobramycin and a newer-generation cephalosporin or a third-generation cephalosporin with *pseudomonas* coverage (see Isaacs' chapter "Medications in the Gastrointestinal Procedure Unit").

Equipment

1. Duodenoscope.
2. Television monitoring system (much preferred) or teaching attachment.
3. Cannulas filled with meglumine diatrizoate (Renografin) diluted to 30% (aids in the detection of small calculi).
4. Fluoroscope with spot film cassettes.
5. Lead aprons and thyroid collars.
6. Gloves and lubricant.

Procedure

1. All personnel must wear lead aprons and thyroid collars.
2. Anesthetize the patient's pharynx with a topical anesthetic.
3. Premedicate the patient with 0.4 mg atropine along with meperidine and midazolam as needed.
4. Pass the side-viewing duodenoscope; inspect the distal esophagus for varices and rapidly examine the stomach.
5. Identify the pylorus and advance the scope to it.
6. When the pylorus is directly in front of the viewing lens, straighten the tip of the scope so that it can pass through the pylorus in its narrowest diameter, neither flexed nor hyperextended. This is accomplished by viewing the top of the pylorus in the 6 o'clock position.
7. Enter the pylorus by advancing the scope, noting the distinct "pop" that may be felt as the duodenum is entered.
8. Inspect the duodenal bulb and then rotate the scope 180° clockwise while simultaneously advancing the scope to enter the descending duodenum.
9. Return the scope to its original upright postion by counterclockwise rotation. At this point, the descending duodenum will be in view. Frequently, the ampulla of Vater will be visible on the medial aspect of the duodenum. If it is not, examine the duodenum until the ampulla is found. Glucagon may be given in 0.2-ml increments to decrease duodenal motility. If the ampulla is not readily found, it is usually because the scope has descended too far into the second part of the duodenum. Retract the scope while looking for the major papilla as well as the minor papillae.
10. When the papilla is identified, roll the patient into the prone position to facilitate cannulation and spot filming.
11. Remove any slack in the duodenoscope by pulling it back. This brings the scope along the lesser curvature of the stomach rather than the greater curvature and will usually improve the angle for cannulation, particularly of the bile duct. This "short-sticking" can be accomplished by placing some clockwise torque on the scope and slowly pulling back, angulating the tip of the scope slightly to keep the ampulla at 12 o'clock. As the scope is pulled back to approximately the 60-cm

level, the ampulla is brought into position by slight movements of the tip of the scope and body torque.

12. Position the ampulla directly in view so that its hood resembles an inverted U with its apex in the 12 o'clock position (Fig. 1). *Do not attempt to cannulate the ampulla until the position is proper.* Any attempt to cannulate without proper orientation usually results in the cannula coming out tangentially. This may produce trauma to the papilla.

13. Once the papilla is properly positioned, cannulate by advancing the catheter by manipulation of the lever control and rotation of the tip of the scope as well as the actual head of the scope. These maneuvers serve to place the tip of the instrument in the proper position. It should be noted that very little movement is necessary during cannulation of the ampulla. Frequent manipulations of the scope, such as advancing and retracting, will lead to patient discomfort and to nausea and vomiting.

14. When the cannula is impacted in the ampulla, advance it for a distance of a few millimeters and inject 1 to 2 cc meglumine diatrizoate.

15. Use fluoroscopy to see which duct is filling.

16. If the pancreatic duct is filling, only 3 to 4 cc dye is needed. Avoid overfilling the pancreatic ductular system. Once lateral branch filling is obtained, stop the injection to *avoid* an acinar pattern. If you are having trouble cannulating the pancreatic duct, remember that it is off to the right of the ampulla and usually toward the bottom and somewhat of a straight shot, compared to the common bile duct whose entrance is on the upper part of the ampulla to the left side and cephalad. Take films of the pancreatic duct in its entirety.

17. Now, turn your attention to filling the other duct, in this case, the common bile duct. Reinsert the cannula and again inject, and if the common bile duct begins to fill, make cer-

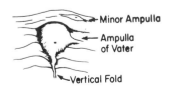

FIG. 1. Major and minor ampulla.

tain that dye is not also going into the pancreatic duct. It may take 15 to 30 cc or more of dye to fill the biliary tree, depending on the presence or absence of the gallbladder. Make certain that no dye enters the pancreatic duct. Placing the patient in a slightly head-down position at this time may be helpful in filling the proximal intrahepatic ducts. If the cannula is seen to be well into the common duct and there is no filling of the pancreatic duct whatsoever, one need not look while injecting dye into the biliary tree except at very infrequent levels. *Remember that fluoroscopic time is high-exposure time—it is hazardous for patient and staff, and damaging to the endoscope.* If difficulty is encountered in entering the common duct selectively, one can attempt to place the cannula tip to the upper left portion of the ampulla and try to bow the cannula so that it takes a cephalad position. Take films of the common bile duct as well as all of the intrahepatic radicles. If small gallstones are suspected, use diluted meglumine diatrizoate (15–30%) as well as a balloon paddle for compression.

18. With good fluoroscopic imaging, it is frequently possible, after having once entered a duct, to know which duct the cannula is in without repeatedly having to inject dye. This avoids overinjection of the pancreatic ductular system.

19. Once films have been obtained and if endoscopic therapy is not necessary, rapidly remove the scope and take additional films. At this time, further positioning, such as placing the patient supine to view the distal common duct and right hepatic system, may be very useful.

Pancreatic Cytology

If pancreatic cytologies are needed, reposition the cannula in the pancreatic duct and give secretin, 1.5 U/kg. Collect pancreatic secretions over 20 min. Several minutes after secretin is given, pancreatic juice will begin to flow and aspiration can be carried out. If fluid does not come, the cannula may be impacted on the wall, and it should be rotated or moved slightly. Collect the pancreatic secretion in two separate vials. The first will contain a few cubic centimeters of meglumine diatrizoate and should be discarded. The remainder of the pancreatic secretion in the second vial is placed on ice and taken to the cytology laboratory for immediate interpretation. Cytologic specimens may also be obtained using catheter-brush assemblies. A radiopaque tip on the cannula may be useful.

Helpful Hints

1. If the cannula will not slip into the puncta, change to a tapered one.
2. "Short-sticking" the duodenoscope, i.e., pulling it back into a position along the lesser curve, is preferred since manipulation of the cannula and cannulation of the common bile duct is easier (Fig. 2A).
3. Frequently, cannulation of the pancreatic duct is more readily accomplished with the scope in a midposition rather than "a short stick."
4. To cannulate the minor ampulla, place the duodenoscope along the greater curvature and use a tapered or metal-tipped cannula (Fig. 2B), designed for minor ampulla cannulation.
5. Do not try to cannulate from too far a distance; get close to the ampulla and use deliberate, small movements to position the endoscope properly.
6. When a periampullary diverticulum is present, look for the ampulla along the edge.
7. If there is difficulty in finding the ampulla of Vater, it is usually because the operator is beyond it in the descending duodenum.
8. If the axis of the ampulla and puncta is not well aligned for cannulation with the patient in the prone position, change the patient's position to the oblique or lateral.
9. Previous duodenal or bile duct surgery may change the anatomy and pliability of the duodenum and impede cannulation.

Postprocedure

1. Monitor vital signs.
2. When the patient's normal pharyngeal function has returned, clear liquids are permitted and then continued for 24 hr.

FIG. 2. Schematic of the endoscope in "short-sticking" (**A**) and for cannulating the minor ampulla (**B**).

3. If there is obstruction to either the pancreatic or the biliary tree and the dye does not drain completely from the pancreatic duct or the common bile duct, start the patient on appropriate antibiotics.

Complications

1. Pancreatitis (0.7–7%).
2. Cholangitis (0.65–0.8%).
3. Duodenal perforation (rare).
4. Hemorrhage (rare).
5. Hyperamylasemia without clincial pancreatitis (commonly seen).

BIBLIOGRAPHY

1. Cryan EM, Falkiner FR, Mulvihill TE, Keane CT, Keeling PW (1984): Pseudomonas aeruginosa cross-infection following endoscopic retrograde cholangiopancreatography. *J Hosp Infect* 5:371–376.
2. Dutta SK, Cox M, Williams RB, Eisenstate TE, Standiford HC (1983): Prospective evaluation of the risk of bacteremia and the role of antibotics in ERCP. *J Clin Gastroenterol* 5:325–329.
3. DiMagno EP, Malagelada JR, Taylor WF, Go VLW (1977): A prospective comparison of current diagnositc tests for pancreatic cancer. *N Engl J Med* 297:737–742.
4. Vennes JA (1977): Technique of ERCP. In: *Atlas of Endoscopic Retrograde Cholangiopancreatography*, edited by ET Stewart, JA Vennes, JE Geenen, pp 4–18. Mosby, St Louis.
5. Bar-Meir S, Greenen JE, et al. (1979): Biliary and pancreatic duct pressures measured by ERCP manometry in patients with suspected papillary stenosis. *Dig Dis Sci* 24:209.
6. Takemoto T, Kasugai T (1979): *Endoscopic Retrograde Cholangiopancreatography*. Igaku-Shoin, Tokyo.
7. Stewart ET, Bennes JA, Geenen JE (1977): *Atlas of Endoscopic Retrograde Cholangiopancreatography*. Mosby, St. Louis.
8. Classen M, Gennen J, Kawai K (1979): *The Papilla Vateri and Its Diseases*. Gerhard Witzstrock Publishing House, New York.
9. Shahml M, Schuman B (1980): Complications of fiberoptic endoscopy. *Gastrointest Endosc* 26:86–91.
10. Neoptolemos JP, Hall AW, Finlay DF, et al (1984): The urgent diagnosis of gallstones in acute pancreatitis: a prospective study of three methods. *Br J Surg* 71:230.

22 / Colonoscopy

Douglas A. Drossman

Colonoscopy involves examination of the colon and terminal ileum by using a fiberoptic or video endoscope. Compared to the gastroscope, the instrument is longer, has a larger instrument channel, and is modified to allow greater torque response. The procedure is technically more difficult, requires more patient preparation, and has a slightly greater complication rate than upper gastrointestinal (GI) endoscopy (1).

Indications

As determined by clinical need, patient condition, and cost-effectiveness:

1. Abnormal barium enema examination that requires further evaluation.
2. Occult lower GI bleeding and/or unexplained iron deficiency anemia.
3. Gross lower GI bleeding that has stabilized.
4. Preoperative or postoperative evaluation of patients with colonic cancer.
5. Screening for colonic neoplasia in high-risk patients (e.g., ulcerative pancolitis for more than 7 years, or left-sided colitis for more than 15 years, family history of polyposis or cancer).
6. Inflammatory bowel disease, radiation, or ischemic colitis that requires assessment of type or extent of disease (e.g., preparation for surgery).
7. Unexplained chronic diarrhea.
8. Therapeutic. Polypectomy, coagulation of bleeding lesions, reduction of volvulus or intussusception, decompression of

atonically distended colon, dilatation of strictures, removal of foreign bodies.
 9. Follow-up evaluation of patients who have had previous polypectomy or surgery for colon carcinoma.

Contraindications
Absolute

1. Peritonitis.
2. Bowel perforation.
3. Toxic or fulminant colitis.
4. Acute diverticulitis.
5. Recent myocardial infarction or pulmonary embolus.

Relative

1. Poor bowel preparation.
2. Inability of patient to physically tolerate or cooperate with the procedure.
3. Recent bowel surgery or history of multiple pelvic operations.
4. Large hernia.
5. Massive colonic bleeding.
6. Unstable cardiopulmonary state (may require monitor and/or respiratory assitance).

Preparation
Bowel Cleansing
Lavage Solution

GoLYTELY (Braintree Laboratories, Inc., Braintree, Massachusetts 02184) or COLYTE (Reed & Carnrick Pharmaceuticals, Jersey City, New Jersey 07302). This has become our standard bowel-cleansing method; it permits excellent visualization, has few side effects, and does not cause dehydration or fluid overload (2). It is contraindicated in patients with possible intestinal obstruction, bowel perforation, toxic colitis, or megacolon.

1. Low-fiber diet for 48 hr prior to colonoscopy.
2. Clear-liquid meal the night before the procedure.
3. 250 cc of prepared solution should be taken orally every 10 to 15 min until at least 1 gallon is consumed. No additional ingredients (e.g., flavorings) should be added to the solution. However, a flavored lavage solution is now available. Alternatively, the solution may be given to the inpatient by nasogastric tube.

Alternate Bowel Preparation

1. Clear fluids for 48 to 72 hr (3,000 cc/day).
2. 60 cc milk of magnesia 2 nights before procedure.
3. 10 oz. p.o. magnesium citrate and tap water enema on night before procedure.
4. Tap water enema until clear on day of procedure.

Inform the patient of the indications for the procedure, alternative therapy, and possible complications. Obtain informed, written consent. Start the intravenous (i.v.) line.

Premedication

See the chapter by Isaacs, "Medications in the Gastrointestinal Procedure Unit," for recommendations regarding subacute bacterial endocarditis (SBE) prophylaxis. Medicate with meperidine, up to 25 to 50 mg i.v., slowly until mild sedation or relaxation is achieved. If needed, administer midazolam (up to 1 mg). Diazepam may produce phlebitis and excessive respiratory depression in elderly or malnourished patients.

Equipment

1. Colonoscope.
2. Light source and video system.
3. Biopsy forceps, washing cannula, and other accessories as needed.
4. Lubricating jelly [or viscous lidocaine (Xylocaine) if perianal inflammation present].
5. Gloves, gauze, and towels.

6. Continuous EKG and/or pulse oximetry as clinically indicated.

Procedure

The following summarizes our use of nonfluoroscopic colonoscopic technique. A more detailed discussion can be found elsewhere (3,4).

1. Position the patient in the left lateral position. The patient's knees should be drawn up with the buttocks at the edge of the examining table.
2. Perform a rectal examination using two sets of gloves.
3. As the finger is withdrawn, guide the lubricated end of the colonoscope over the finger and advance 3 to 4 cm into the rectum.
4. Remove the outer gloves to avoid greasing the head of the scope.
5. Many endoscopists keep the left-right control partially locked throughout the procedure to maintain torque stability at the tip of the scope.
6. Control tip deflection and scope passage with the right hand grasping the insertion tube near the anus. Remove the hand only to reposition the left-right controls at the head of the scope.
7. Let the colonoscope hang toward the floor with the right thigh bracing the insertion tube (at about 20 cm from the anus) against the table. This prevents the scope from slipping out of the rectum when the right hand is removed and "shortens" the scope length to permit easier passage control.
8. Position the left hand on the head of the scope so that the thumb can freely move the up-down controls.
9. Visualize the rectum. Usually, a "red-out" is first seen; withdraw the instrument 1 to 2 cm and insufflate air until the mucosa and lumen are seen.
10. Advance the scope under direct visualization, directing the tip as much as possible with torque maneuvers by the right hand. Advancing the scope along the lesser curve of the bowel lumen tends to minimize loop formation.

11. Use of torque. This is a technique for advancing the scope around bends. It causes stiffening of the tube and, with the controls locked, also turns the tip of the scope. In the region of the sigmoid, a counterclockwise spiral is usually made. After that, lesser degrees of clockwise torque are needed to get around the flexures. When the lumen angulates behind a fold, torque the scope so the tip turns into the lumen and advance it.
12. Relubricate the anal area whenever resistance occurs.
13. *Technique in difficult situations.* When uncertain of what to do or where the scope tip is located, make frequent use of withdrawing movements. When no lumen is seen, withdraw and "jiggle." A jiggle is a series of rapid in-and-out movements with torque directed toward the lumen. If a crescent is seen indicating lumen behind it, turn the scope into the crescent and jiggle while gradually withdrawing. This sheaths the bowel on the scope, straightens it, and tends to move the lumen into view (Fig. 1). *Do not* advance (push) if a loop is being made (determined by paradoxical movement or less than a 1:1 response of the tip-to-tube passage from the rectum), if you cannot see lumen, or if resistance to passage occurs. In these situations, the following maneuvers may be tried:
    a. Jiggle the tube.
    b. Straighten the tube by withdrawing.
    c. Change the position of the patient. For example, place the patient in the right lateral position to traverse the splenic flexure, or supine to traverse the hepatic flexure.
    d. Suck out air. This tends to shorten the bowel and advance the tip. This is most successful on the right side of the colon.
    e. Apply abdominal pressure. Downward pressure on the sigmoid colon loop in the left lower quadrant tends to straighten it. Upward midabdominal pressure straightens the transverse colon. Lifting up the right pelvic abdomen can help advance the scope into the cecum when it will not progress beyond the ileocecal valve.
    f. In some cases, pushing through the loop may afford progress ("slide-by"), although it produces greater patient discomfort.

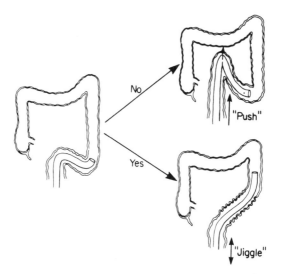

FIG. 1. Techniques for advancing the endoscope in difficult situations. Pushing the endoscope through areas of angulation tends to form loops. A series of gentle but rapid in-and-out motions sheaths the colon on the endoscope and tends to straighten the bowel, thus permitting advancement.

14. Remain aware of intracolonic landmarks:
    a. The *rectum* has prominent bluish vessels. The semilunar valves of Houston are usually seen best on withdrawal of the instrument.
    b. The *rectosigmoid angulus* occurs at about 15 to 17 cm.
    c. The *sigmoid colon* has concentric and symmetric ring-like valvulae.
    d. The *descending colon* is long and tubular in appearance; the valvulae may be absent.
    e. The dome of the *splenic flexure* is seen at the proximal end of the descending colon. Occasionally, the bluish impression of the spleen is seen. The transverse colon is entered after a sharp angulation.
    f. The *transverse colon* has large, thin triangular folds formed by the lateral muscle bands, the taeniae coli. Light transmitted from the scope in the transverse colon may be seen anywhere on the abdomen.
    g. The *hepatic flexure* is seen just after the liver imparts a bluish appearance to the proximal transverse colon. The

flexure traverses posteriorly and downward for about 10 cm and will transilluminate the patient's right flank.
 h. The *ascending colon* has asymmetric folds, and the lumen is quite large. It will illuminate the right upper and lower abdominal quadrants.
 i. The *cecum* can be identified when
  i. The light is transmitted through the skin just above the right inguinal ligament.
  ii. The terminal ileum, appendiceal lumen, and sling fold of the caput cecum ("Mercedes Benz" sign) are identified.
  iii. A lumen cannot be visualized (least reliable).
 j. Sometimes, pushing with one finger on the abdomen and noting the area of greatest indentation through the scope is helpful.
15. *Cannulation of the ileum.* The ileocecal valve is not well visualized, as it is directed downward into the cecum (Fig. 2A). It is usually found medially behind a flat, rolled fold located just before entering the cecum and 3 cm above the terminal portion of the cecum. Cannulation is best accomplished by advancing the scope beyond the fold, turning into the fold, and slowly withdrawing the scope while gently torquing the shaft back and forth (Fig. 2B). Often the tip will "pop" through the valve, and it can then be advanced into the ileum (Fig. 2C).
16. Perform a thorough examination of the colon when withdrawing from the cecum. *This is the most important part of the procedure.* Check behind folds and examine carefully the lesser curvatures. The natural tendency on withdrawing is for the scope to straighten, thereby visualizing mainly the greater curvatures.
17. When the rectum is reached, the endoscope can be retroflexed to examine for hemorrhoids, papillitis, fissures, or other anorectal disorders.

Postprocedure

Be certain that the patient's condition is stable. Write a brief postprocedure note in the medical record containing the following:

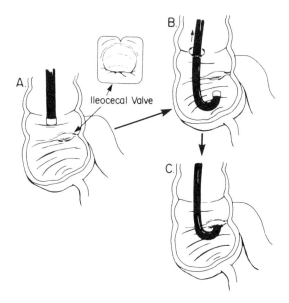

FIG. 2. Cannulation of the ileocecal valve. The valve orifice is directed downward and away from the endoscope. Cannulation can be accomplished by (**A**) advancing the endoscope beyond the fold, (**B**) turning into the fold and slowly withdrawing the scope while gently torquing the shaft back and forth. The tip will "pop" through the valve and advance into the ileum (**C**).

1. Indications for procedure.
2. Type of instrument used.
3. The visual level reached.
4. Medication given.
5. Procedures done (e.g., biopsy, cytology).
6. Adequacy of prep and difficulties encountered (e.g., excessive pain or bleeding, poor visualization).
7. Clinical findings.
8. Postprocedure condition of the patient.
9. Follow-up plan.

REFERENCES

1. Silvis SE, Nebel O, Rogers G, Sugawa C, Mandelstam P (1976): Endoscopic complications. Results of the 1974 American Society for Gastrointestinal Endoscopy survey. *JAMA* 235:928–930.

2. Ernstoff JJ, Howard DA, Marshall JB, Jumshyd A, McCullough AJ (1983): A randomized blinded clinical trial of a rapid colonic lavage solution (Golytely) compared with standard preparation for colonoscopy and barium enema. *Gastroenterology* 84:1512–1516.
3. Waye JD (1981): Colonoscopy intubation techniques without fluoroscopy. In: *Colonoscopy. Techniques, Clinical Practice and Colour Atlas*, edited by RH Hunt, JD Waye, pp 147–178. Chapman and Hall, London.
4. Williams CB, Waye JD (1991): Colonoscopy and flexible sigmoidoscopy. In: *Textbook of Gastroenterology*, edited by T Yamada, DH Alpers, C Dwyang, DW Powell, FE Silverstein, pp 2249–2265. JB Lippincott Company, Philadelphia.

23 / Flexible Sigmoidoscopy

Robert S. Sandler

The flexible sigmoidoscope is a fiberoptic or video endoscope designed to examine the rectum and sigmoid colon. The instrument was developed in order to correct several of the deficiencies of the rigid sigmoidoscope. It was thought that the flexibility of the instrument would provide patients with a more comfortable exam and that the longer length would detect more lesions. These goals have generally been met. Patients report less discomfort, anxiety, and embarrassment during flexible as compared to rigid sigmoidoscopy (1). The flexible instrument has been shown to detect a significantly greater number of malignant and premalignant lesions (2). Many regard the flexible sigmoidoscope as the primary diagnostic instrument for examination of the rectosigmoid.

Indications

The general indication for flexible sigmoidoscopy is to search for abnormalities within reach of the instrument. Specific indications include:

1. Screening. The precise role of sigmoidoscopy in screening asymptomatic adults has not been established (3). Although some North American health organizations recommend periodic sigmoidoscopies, others make no recommendations for or against the procedure (4).
2. Minor bright-red rectal bleeding. Although the flexible sigmoidoscope will not localize bleeding below 20 cm any better than the rigid scope, it may reveal other pathology in the rectosigmoid above the reach of the rigid instrument. Bleed-

ing from an anal fissure or internal hemorrhoid is easily missed, so anoscopy should also be employed to evaluate patients with bright-red rectal bleeding. Unexplained lower gastrointestinal bleeding or iron deficiency anemia requires full colonoscopy.

3. To evaluate symptoms of acute or chronic diarrhea, rectal pain, tenesmus, constipation, or change in bowel habits.
4. To reduce a sigmoid volvulus.
5. To examine anastomoses for stricture, bleeding, or recurrent tumor.
6. Inflammatory bowel disease. To monitor disease activity when full colonoscopy is not needed; to evaluate patients with acute colitis.
7. Adjunct to X-ray. To evaluate lesions seen on X-ray within reach of the instrument; to examine a tortuous rectosigmoid where lesions can be missed on X-ray.
8. Physical incapacity. The lateral position used for flexible sigmoidoscopy is well suited for the elderly and those with debilitating illnesses, cardiac decompensation, or broken limbs.
9. Pseudomembranous colitis. The characteristic 2- to 5-mm, yellow-white raised plaques scattered over the mucosal surface can be readily seen and biopsied (5).

Contraindications

The contraindications to flexible sigmoidoscopy are to some extent relative. They must be balanced against the potential information that the study can provide.

1. Acute peritonitis.
2. Fulminant colitis/toxic megacolon.
3. Uncooperative patient.
4. Acute, severe diverticulitis.

Preparation

1. A single Fleet (or other proprietary small-volume hypertonic phosphate) enema given 5 to 20 min prior to the exam will provide adequate preparation in 80% to 90% of cases. Outpa-

tients may take the enema at home 1 to 2 hr before the procedure.
2. Obtain informed written consent.
3. The exam is usually performed without sedation.
4. Endocarditis prophylaxis: See the chapter by Isaacs, "Medications in the Gastrointestinal Procedure Unit."

Equipment

1. Flexible sigmoidoscope. There are a number of instruments available.
2. Light source.
3. Suction.
4. Biopsy forceps, cytology brush.
5. Gloves.
6. Lubricant.
7. Gown for patient and operator.
8. Permit form, result sheet.
9. Water for irrigation.
10. Luer-tip syringe, 50 cc.

Procedure

The technique of flexible sigmoidoscopy is similar to that of colonoscopy (see the chapter by Drossman, "Colonoscopy"). Excellent descriptions of the technique appear in the literature (6). Although there are both plastic and computer simulation models available for training, there is no substitute for hands-on training under the supervision of a skilled endoscopist.

1. Place the patient in the left lateral decubitus position.
2. Do a careful rectal exam. If stool is encountered, administer another enema.
3. Examine the anal canal and distal rectum with an anoscope before sigmoidoscopy in patients with symptoms localized to the anal area.
4. Lubricate the distal 10 to 15 cm of the instrument. Do not get lubricant on the lens. Make sure that the air and suction are operating adequately.
5. Insert the instrument into the anus as the gloved finger is

withdrawn or gently insert the tube obliquely by pressing the curved surface of the tip against the sphincter, rather than straight on (Fig. 1).

6. On entry to the rectum there is usually a "red-out" indicating that the tip abuts the mucosa. Apply gentle bursts of air, withdraw the scope, and angulate the tip to locate the lumen. The tip should constantly be maneuvered to keep the lumen in view as the instrument is advanced. Use as little air as possible. Air distension stretches the colon, making the exam more difficult and more uncomfortable for the patient.

7. When the lumen is not seen, pull the scope back a few centimeters. The pattern of folds as the bowel collapses behind the withdrawing endoscope will indicate the proper direction of passage. If the colon is in spasm, as indicated by puckered folds, apply gentle bursts of air to distend the lumen. In advancing the scope, steer toward the dark center of the lumen.

8. For the beginner, simply advance the tube until it will go no further with gentle pressure. Technical maneuvers to advance the scope further should be reserved for those with more experience. The goal is to provide a safe, thorough, and comfortable exam and not to insert the instrument to its

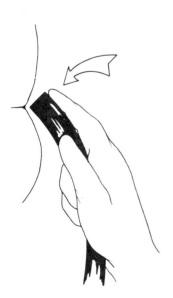

FIG. 1. Correct 90° wedged insertion.

full length. Stubborn attempts to insert the scope risk harming the patient.

9. If the tube will not advance around the rectosigmoid junction (at about 15 cm), gentle pressure will sometimes open the angle and permit the scope to pass. This maneuver is safe, even if the lumen is not clearly seen ahead, as long as the mucosa slides by. If the patient is uncomfortable, or if the scope does not advance, withdraw and try rotating the shaft of the scope (torque).

10. Torque may be applied with short scopes by rotating the control head of the instrument, and with longer scopes by twisting the shaft itself near the anus. Gentle clockwise torque is often effective to help advance the scope, find the lumen, and straighten angulated bowel. By pulling the scope back while applying torque, loops in the bowel can be straightened.

11. Moving the tube in and out a few centimeters at a time (jiggling, dithering) may also sleeve the bowel onto the scope. This maneuver, which is often effectively combined with torque, is described in greater detail in the chapter by Drossman, "Colonoscopy."

12. The bowel is best examined on slow withdrawal of the instrument. The tip should be methodically deflected behind each valve and fold. Air insufflation, torque, and tip deflection can be used on withdrawal.

13. Endoscopic pinch biopsies should be taken of any lesions seen. Diminutive polyps (< 5 mm) should be biopsied to determine whether they are adenomatous or hyperplastic. We do not believe that finding hyperplastic polyps in the rectosigmoid demands full colonoscopy (7), but this is controversial.

14. To prevent explosions, coagulation biopsies (hot biopsies) or snare electrocautery should not be attempted unless the patient has had a full colonoscopic prep.

Postprocedure

1. Review the findings with the patient.
2. The patient may resume normal activities immediately.

3. If biopsy specimens were taken, caution the patient that small quantities of blood may be seen in the stool.

REFERENCES

1. Winawer SJ, Miller C, Lightdale C, et al (1987): Patient response to sigmoidoscopy: a randomized, controlled trial of rigid and flexible sigmiodoscopy. *Cancer* 60:1905–1908.
2. Wilking N, Petrelli NJ, Herrera-Ornelas L, Walsh D, Mittelman A (1986): A comparison of the 25-cm rigid proctosigmoidoscope with the 65-cm flexible endoscope in the screening of patients for colorectal carcinoma. *Cancer* 57:669–671.
3. Selby JV, Friedman GD (1989): Sigmoidoscopy in the periodic health examination of asymptomatic adults. *JAMA* 261:595–601.
4. Hayward RSA, Steinberg EP, Ford DE, Roizen MF, Roach KW (1991): Preventive care guidelines: 1991. *Ann Intern Med* 114:758–783.
5. LaMont T (1991): Bacterial infections of the colon. In: *Textbook of Gastroenterology*, edited by T Yamada, p 1758. JB Lippincott Company, Philadelphia.
6. Katon RM, Keefe EB, Melnyk CS (1985): *Flexible Sigmoidoscopy*. Grune & Stratton, Orlando.
7. Provenzale D, Garrett JW, Condon SE, Sandler RS (1990): Risk for colon adenomas in patients with rectosigmoid hyperplastic polyps. *Ann Intern Med* 113:760–763.

24 / Anoscopy and Rigid Sigmoidoscopy

Don W. Powell

The increased use of flexible sigmoidoscopy to examine the rectum and distal colon has not alleviated the need for the physician to become proficient in the use of the anoscope and rigid sigmoidoscope. Most gastroenterologists believe that the anal canal is still most optimally evaluated with the anoscope. Anoscopy and rigid sigmoidoscopy are still convenient methods if the physician is only interested in the distal 15 cm of the alimentary canal (e.g., when considering hemorrhoids or proctitis as a cause of rectal bleeding, following the disease course of patients with known proctitis, or when evaluating the anorectum for conditions such as fistula in ano or perirectal abscess). In addition, rigid sigmoidoscopy can be performed anywhere there is an electrical outlet, with largely disposable equipment that does not require expertise for cleaning or maintenance, and without the need for specially trained ancillary personnel. To ensure the most complete examination of the colorectum and the anus, anoscopy could be performed in conjunction with either flexible sigmoidoscopy or colonoscopy.

Indications (1–5)

1. Symptoms referable to the colon, rectum, or anus: bleeding, discharge, protrusions or swellings, abdominal or anorectal pain, diarrhea, constipation or a change in bowel habits, severe itching.
2. Unexplained fever.
3. Patient evaluation prior to anorectal surgery (flexible sigmoidoscopy is preferred).

4. To observe the progression or regression of colorectal disease.
5. To obtain tissue for histologic study or stool and/or exudate for bacteriologic or parasitologic study.
6. To remove foreign bodies from the rectum.
7. To evaluate the rectum in any patient in whom a barium enema is to be performed.
8. As a routine part of the physical examination, although the age at which this is to begin and the frequency of such an examination, as well as the cost-effectiveness, remain controversial.

Contraindications

There are no absolute contraindications to proctosigmoidoscopy.

1. Because patients with heart disease have an increase in ectopic beats with sigmoidoscopy, cardiac monitoring and/or awareness of possible arrhythmias in these patients are advised (6).
2. Because bacteremia occurs in 10% of patients undergoing sigmoidoscopy (7), antibiotic prophylaxis (including coverage for the enterococcus) is advised in patients with valvular or congenital heart disease who are at risk (see the chapter by Isaacs, "Medications in the Gastrointestinal Procedure Unit").

Preparation

1. Most patients can and should be examined with no prior preparation.
2. If stool precludes an adequate examination, a bisacodyl suppository or Fleet enema can be given and the examination carried out 1 hr later.
3. In rare circumstances, a tap water or saline solution enema given at bedtime the night before and then repeated the next morning 3 to 4 hr prior to examination will be necessary for optimal visualization.
4. Premedication (sedation) is rarely necessary, although intra-

venous meperidine and/or diazepam can be useful in unusual circumstances.

Equipment

Minimal Equipment

1. An anoscope and sigmoidoscope. An adult sigmoidoscope is adequate for all but the infant.
2. Cotton swab sticks.
3. An examination table or bed.
4. A sheet to cover the patient.
5. Gloves, lubricant, and 4 × 4 in. gauze pads.

Useful Equipment

1. Sigmoidoscopy table.
2. Suction.
3. Air insufflator.
4. Sigmoidoscopy spoon.
5. Biopsy tools: either alligator type (see Procedure section, Rectal Biopsy with Alligator Forceps), colonoscopic biopsy forceps taped to a stick, or suction-type biopsy capsule.
6. Epinephrine solution and silver nitrate sticks.

Procedure

Be gentle and reassuring throughout the procedure. Inform the patient what is to be done. Advise the patient that a few deep breaths during the examination will often relax muscles and sphincters.

Position

Position the patient for the examination (2,3).

Left Lateral (Sims') Position

This is best for bedridden or feeble patients or to assess anal pathology such as hemorrhoids. Be sure to get buttocks to the edge of the bed or table by placing the patient diagionally across the bed (Fig. 1a).

Knee-Chest Position

This is adequate for most examinations. It requires more patient stamina and cooperation (Fig. 1b).

Prone, Inverted (Jackknife) Position with Sigmoidoscopy Table

This is the most comfortable position for the patient and the examiner (Fig. 1c). Place the patient's knee rest high enough so that the "broken" table does not compress the abdomen. This allows the pelvic organs to "fall away" when the sigmoidoscope is advanced. Elbow rests are preferred so that the patient does not slide off the end of the table (Fig. 1d).

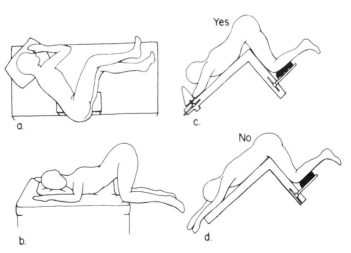

FIG. 1. Three major positions for anoscopy and sigmoidoscopy. **a:** Left lateral (Sims') position. **b:** Knee-chest position. **c:** Prone, inverted (jackknife) position. **d:** An improper jackknife position is shown; the knee rest is too low, and no elbow rest is provided.

Digital Examination

Inspect the perianal area and perform a digital examination (8).

1. If two gloves are worn on the examining hand, some decrease in sensitivity of touch is experienced; but time is saved, since the soiled glove can be stripped off, and one can proceed with anoscopy or sigmoidoscopy.
2. Spread the buttocks apart and inspect the perineum for cutaneous or anal pathology.
3. Palpate the perianal and perineal tissues for abscesses or fistulae.
4. Perform the digital exam with a well-lubricated finger. The digital exam relaxes the anal sphincters and facilitates insertion of the scope. Try to palpate any abnormalities you wish to visualize at anoscopy. Sweep the finger circumferentially around the anal canal; a blind spot to sigmoidoscopy is directly posterior and proximal to the anal ring. Examine anteriorly for cul-de-sac lesions; do not mistake the cervix for tumor. Stool from the examining finger can be checked for occult blood.

Anoscopic Examination

Perform anoscopic examination (4–6). The anoscope is most useful to view fissures, fistula openings, internal hemorrhoids, papillitis and cryptitis, and neoplasm.

1. Insert a clean plastic anoscope. It should be warm and well lubricated.
2. Stabilize the obturator with the thumb and insert by aiming toward the umbilicus.
3. After inserting 3 to 4 cm, move the tip posteriorly.
4. If anal spasm is encountered, ask the patient to bear down or breathe through the mouth.
5. Visual examination of hemorrhoids with the anoscope is facilitated by having the patient strain (Valsalva) as you remove the anoscope. This is particularly important in the knee-chest position, where internal hemorrhoids may collapse.

Sigmoidoscopy Examination

Perform sigmoidoscopic examination (4–6).

1. Introduce the sigmoidoscope blindly only for the first 3 to 5 cm while stabilizing the obturator with the thumb. Aim toward the umbilicus (Fig. 2a). Remove the obturator and, from this point on, advance the sigmoidoscope under direct vision.
2. Swing the tip of the sigmoidoscope posteriorly to follow the curve of the sacrum (Fig. 2b). Advance the scope as far as possible.
3. If the lumen is lost, the end of the sigmoidoscope is probably occluded by a valve or the rectal wall or is at the rectosigmoid junction (Fig. 2c). Do not push forward! Pull back 2 to 3 cm, rotate the scope until the lumen reappears, and then advance (Fig. 2d). Often, the tip of the advancing scope can

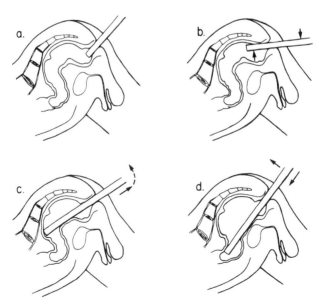

FIG. 2. Sequence of steps of the sigmoidoscopy. **a:** Sigmoidoscope, with obturator, is inserted, aimed toward the umbilicus. **b:** With the obturator removed, the tip of the scope is rotated posteriorly and advanced. **c:** If the lumen is lost, the sigmoidoscope is retracted until the lumen is found and (**d**) then advanced.

"iron out" a fold or curve and aid in passage. Some examiners insufflate air if the lumen cannot be visualized; however, this may produce some discomfort. The rectosigmoid junction is encountered at 12 to 15 cm, and many sigmoidoscopies will end here. Often, this point can be negotiated by straightening the bend with the end of the scope or by insufflating air.

4. Withdraw the scope slowly, rotating the tip circumferentially to observe the entire rectal wall. Check the stool from this point for occult blood. Also test the mucosa for friability. Twirl a swab on the mucosa; then remove it and observe for capillary bleeding. Look behind the rectal valves of Houston.

Rectal Biopsy with Alligator Forceps

1. Unless a specific lesion is to be biopsied, the posterior rectal mucosa should be biopsied below the peritoneal reflection (within 7–10 cm of the anal verge) to lessen the chance of free peritoneal perforation.
2. Biopsies from the free edge of a valve are technically the easiest, but the large biopsy obtained increases the chance of bleeding or perforation. Biopsy from the base of the valve is probably safer.
3. Bleeding can usually be stopped by applying pressure with a dry cotton or with epinephrine-soaked swabs (1 ml of 1:1,000 epinephrine diluted 1 to 10 with saline fluid).
4. After the bleeding has halted, the biopsy site may be cauterized with silver nitrate sticks.

Postprocedure

The patient may resume normal activity. Inform the patient that some "gas pains" may be experienced, but to notify you if persistent pain or bleeding occurs.

REFERENCES

1. Schrock TR (1978): Examination of the anorectum, sigmoidoscopy, and colonoscopy. In: *Gastrointestinal Disease: Pathophysiology, Diagnosis,*

Management, 2nd ed, edited by MH Sleisenger, JS Fordtran, pp 1548–1559. WB Saunders Company, Philadelphia.

2. Goligher JC, Duthie HL, Nixon HH (1980): *Surgery of the Anus, Rectum, and Colon*. Bailliére Tindall, London.

3. Otto P, Ewe K (1979): *Atlas of Rectoscopy and Colonoscopy*. Springer-Verlag, Berlin.

4. Turell R (1960): Proctosigmoidoscopy. *The New Physician* 9:23–28.

5. Castro AF (1960): Diagnosis and management of common rectal and anal disorders. *Am Fam Physician* 34:78–92.

6. Fletcher GF, Earnest DL, Shuford WF, Wenger NK (1968): Electrocardiographic changes during routine sigmoidoscopy. *Arch Intern Med* 122:483–486.

7. LeFrock JL, Ellis CA, Truchik JB, Weinstein L (1973): Transient bacteremia associated with sigmoidoscopy. *N Engl J Med* 289:467–470.

8. Barnett JL, Raper SE (1991): Anorectal diseases. In: *Textbook of Gastroenterology*, edited by T Yamada, DH Alpers, C Owyang, DW Powell, FE Silverstein, pp 1813–1835. JB Lippincott Company, Philadelphia.

25 / Dilatation of the Esophagus: Mercury-Filled Bougies (Hurst-Maloney)

Eugene M. Bozymski

Esophageal stricture is a severe complication of gastroesophageal reflux and, once established, is difficult to manage in an entirely satisfactory manner. One of the mainstays in treating such strictures, as well as other entities that obliterate the esophageal lumen, is periodic dilatation. The oldest, least expensive, and still frequently used method is the use of mercury-filled bougies of graded sizes. Two main types are available: the blunt rounded Hurst dilators and the tapered Maloney dilators (Fig. 1).

Indications

1. Peptic esophageal strictures.
2. Caustic strictures.
3. Radiation-induced strictures.
4. Palliation for esophageal carcinoma.
5. Upper esophageal webs.
6. Lower esophageal rings.
7. Occasionally for diffuse esophageal spasm with significant dysphagia.

Contraindications

1. Significant bleeding diathesis.
2. Recent (within 10–14 days) esophageal biopsies, particularly those obtained with a Rubin-Quinton multipurpose suction biopsy tube.

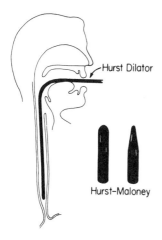

Hurst Dilator

Hurst-Maloney

FIG. 1. Hurst dilator being passed through esophageal stricture.

3. Impacted bolus.
4. Lack of patient cooperation.
5. Recent myocardial infarction.
6. Esophageal diverticulum.
7. Severe cervical arthritis.

Preparation

1. Obtain prior radiologic and/or endoscopic evaluation of the upper gastrointestinal tract.
2. If the stricture is so severe that caloric intake has been markedly impaired, hospitalize the patient and perform the dilatations over several days.
3. Nothing by mouth for 8 hr.
4. Obtain informed, written consent.
5. Anesthetize the pharynx with a topical agent, such as Cetacaine or Hurricaine.
6. Very *infrequently*, the patient may need preprocedure sedation with midazolam or meperidine.
7. If the patient has a prosthetic valve in place, one should follow the recommendations of the American Heart Association with respect to antibiotic therapy (see the chapter by Isaacs, "Medications in the Gastrointestinal Procedure Unit").

Equipment

1. Hurst and Maloney dilators.
2. Gloves, basin, gowns, and towels.
3. Lubricant.
4. Fluoroscopic equipment should be available, since confirmation of dilator position is occasionally necessary.

Procedure

1. The Hurst dilator with its blunt end should be the initial bougie used for most strictures of the esophagus. Maloney dilators with their tapered end are often used for longer strictures because the tapered end serves as a lumen finder.
2. Start with the size most appropriate, based on the previous endoscopic examination or a prior dilatation. For example, if the stricture was judged to be 6 mm in transverse diameter on endoscopic exam, an 18 French Hurst bougie should be used as the initial dilator (1 mm is roughly equivalent to 3 French). If the patient was dilated to 30 French 1 week earlier, it would be appropriate to start the subsequent dilatation with the same-size bougie.
3. Seat the patient lower than the operator and place the dilator in the posterior pharynx, resting it on the cricopharyngeus.
4. Ask the patient to swallow.
5. Pass the tube while the nurse assists by keeping the weighted column of mercury above the patient's head.
6. If passage through the stricture is difficult, it often helps to place the volar surface of the index and middle fingers of the left hand against the hard palate to anchor the bougie in place while exerting mild pressure with the right hand on the bougie. Most often a "pop" or a "give" can be felt as the stricture is passed. Also, greater resistance is noted when pulling the dilator back through the stricture.
7. Dilatations are usually carried out with three dilators, depending on the ease of the procedure and patient tolerance. Stop the dilatation at the point where blood is noted on the dilator or if the patient complains of severe pain.

8. Redilate the stricture within a few days, starting with size of the last dilator from the previous dilatation. If it will not pass, drop back a size or two and work up again.
9. With short strictures, larger dilators may at times pass more easily, whereas smaller dilators will be too flimsy. Proceed with caution.
10. Fluoroscopic confirmation is necessary when there is a question as to whether the bougie is passing through the stricture. At times, the bougie may simply curl in the esophagus or push the esophagus ahead and not pass the stricture.
11. Endoscopic biopsy specimens are usually obtained 10 to 14 days prior to the first dilatation to exclude a neoplastic stricture; however, when the stricture precludes adequate nutritional intake, dilatation should be performed. Brush cytology specimens should be obtained prior to the procedure. Once the stricture is dilated sufficiently to allow passage of the endoscope, complete examination of the esophagus along with biopsies can be accomplished.
12. With dilatation of a lower esophageal ring (Schatzki's ring), two methods have been recommended. One approach is to use graded French Hurst dilators and progress from 32 to 36 to 40 or 42 to 44 to 48. This allows one to stretch as well as rupture the mucosal ring. The other approach is to begin dilatation with one large (44–50 French) bougie.

Postprocedure

1. Most often, the procedures described in this chapter are done on an outpatient basis. The physician must advise the patient to notify him or her immediately if there is chest or back pain, fever, regurgitation, or vomiting of blood.
2. The patient should take nothing by mouth until the anesthetic agent wears off. This can be tested by having the patient attempt to swallow small quantities of water 1 hr after the procedure has been completed.
3. Administer antacids or sucralfate slurry for 4 to 5 days following the procedure. An H_2 receptor antagonist may be appropriate.

Complications

1. Esophageal perforation (< 0.01%).
2. Hemorrhage (< 0.04%).
3. Aspiration.
4. Bacteremia.

BIBLIOGRAPHY

1. Rosenow EC (1974): Techniques of esophageal dilatation. In: *The Esophagus*, edited by WS Payne, AM Olsen, pp 55–64. Lea and Febiger, Philadelphia.
2. Patterson DJ, Graham DY, Smith JL, et al. (1983): Natural history of benign esophageal stricture treated by dilatation. *Gastroenterology* 85:346–350.
3. Welsh JD, Griffiths WJ, McKee J, Wilkinson D, Flournoy DJ, Mohr JA (1983): Bacteremia associated with esophageal dilatation. *J Clin Gastroenterol* 5:109–112.
4. Tulman AB, Boyce HW Jr (1981): Complications of esophageal dilation and guidelines for their prevention. *Gastrointest Endosc* 27:229–234.

26 / Dilatation of the Esophagus: Wire-Guided Bougies (Eder-Puestow and Savary-Gilliard)

Eugene M. Bozymski

Dilatation of very narrow strictures can be carried out by passing bougies of various sizes over previously passed guide wires. A wire with a flexible spring tip can be substituted for the guide wire. This latter system represents the Eder-Puestow wire-guided method of dilating the esophagus and is very useful for initiating dilatation of tight strictures through which a mercury-filled bougie will not pass. The Eder-Puestow system includes a flexible wire with a coiled spring tip (which can be passed through the biopsy channel of an endoscope), a set of olive dilators of various calibers, and a flexible steel pusher rod to which the various dilators can be screwed. The entire assembly then can be passed over the previously passed flexible wire, which serves as a guide wire. The obvious advantage to such a system is that the dilating olive must follow the wire and cannot stray within the lumen, thus decreasing the chance of perforation.

Savary-Gilliard dilators are centrally drilled tapered dilators of varying sizes which are passed over a special spring-tipped guide that is generally placed into the stomach during endoscopy and its position is then confirmed fluoroscopically. The dilatation itself is then carried out in much the same manner as described above. These dilators have achieved a preeminent place in our endoscopy unit and are frequently used in a variety of clinical settings. The Savary-Gilliard system appears to be easier and safer than the Eder-Puestow dilators.

We are also now using a wide array of polyethylene balloon dilators, passed directly through the biopsy channel of the endoscope or over an endoscopically placed tiny flexible 0.035 mm guide wire, in the management of esophageal strictures, and this technique is discussed in the chapter by Heizer, "Balloon Dilatation of Strictures." The choice of which dilator to use in the management of esophageal strictures is dependent on various factors such as lumen size, length of stricture, and operator experience.

Indications

Puestow dilatation is used for strictures that are too small to be dilated with mercury-filled bougies [see chapter by Bozymski, "Dilatation of the Esophagus: Mercury-Filled Bougies (Hurst-Maloney)"].

Contraindications

1. See the chapter by Bozymski, "Dilatation of the Esophagus: Mercury-Filled Bougies (Hurst-Maloney)."
2. Esophageal ulcer.

Preparation

1. Check the hematocrit, platelet count, prothrombin time (PT), and partial thromboplastin time (PTT).
2. Review cervical spine films (if previously obtained) for arthritis.
3. Obtain written, informed consent.
4. Administer topical anesthetic to pharynx.
5. Start an intravenous (i.v.) line for administration of atropine, midazolam, or meperidine as necessary.

Equipment

1. Endoscope (recommended for first dilatation).
2. Wire-guided bougie system (Eder-Puestow and/or Savary-Gilliard).

3. Fluoroscope.
4. Lubricant and gloves.

Procedure

1. Perform endoscopy prior to the first dilatation. This will allow observation of any anatomic esophageal variation, such as the presence of pseudodiverticula or true diverticula, as well as any tortuosity or eccentrically located strictures. If an ulcer is identified, dilatation should be postponed until an antireflux program reduces the inflammation.
2. During direct observation at endoscopy, place the guide wire through the stricture well into the stomach. Pull the endoscope out 5 cm at a time while advancing the wire 5 cm so that the wire tip will remain in position in the stomach.
3. On removal of the endoscope, check the wire position fluoroscopically to make certain that the tip remains in the stomach, well below the stricture.
4. Oral passage of the guide wire without endoscopy may be performed in patients undergoing repeated dilatation. This can be accomplished by having the patient swallow a shortened tube of any type and advancing the guide wire through it. The position of the wire in the stomach must be confirmed by fluoroscopy.
5. Begin the dilatation by passing the most appropriate (dependent on stricture size) olive or Savary dilator over the wire.
6. Gently advance the olive or dilator into the body of the esophagus through the posterior pharynx and cricopharyngeus. Advance the dilator over the guide wire for short distances at a time, maintaining good control by holding the dilator close to the patient's mouth and advancing slowly (Fig. 1).
7. As the stricture is reached, increased resistance is noted and more pressure may be needed to pass through the stricture.
8. Successful passage of the dilator through the stricture should be confirmed fluoroscopically.
9. After the dilator has passed the stricture and one begins to pull it back, the resistance of the stricture will again be felt as the dilator passes through it.

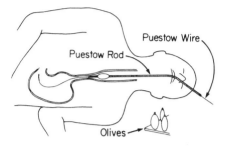

FIG. 1. Puestow wire in place with flexible tip in the stomach. The dilating olive is advanced through the stricture with the Puestow rod.

10. Retrieve the dilator by pulling it back over the guide wire in short, 2- to 5-cm segments.
11. Continue with three progressive dilatations or until blood is noted on the dilator, whereupon the procedure is terminated.
12. Subsequent dilatations can, at times, be performed by passing the wire through the mouth into the stomach under fluoroscopic control. Endoscopic placement is not necessary prior to every dilatation unless one encounters problems. However, fluoroscopic confirmation of the wire placement is always necessary prior to undertaking a dilatation.

Postprocedure

1. See the chapter by Bozymski, "Dilatation of the Esophagus: Mercury-Filled Bougies (Hurst-Maloney)."
2. Monitor vital signs.
3. Elevate the head of the bed.
4. Clear liquids for 24 hr; then if clinically stable, soft diet for 2 days; then routine diet.
5. Antacids, 30 cc between meals and at bedtime for 5 days. Sucralfate 1 g q.i.d. for 5 days is an alternative or H_2 receptor antagonist therapy.

Complications

1. Esophageal perforation (0.3%).
2. Hemorrhage (< 0.1%).

3. Aspiration.
4. Bacteremia.

BIBLIOGRAPHY

1. Rosenow EC (1874): Techniques of esophageal dilatation. In: *The Esophagus*, edited by WS Payne, AM Olsen, pp 55–64. Lea and Febiger, Philadelphia.
2. Mandelstam P, Sugawa C, Silvis SE, Nebel OT, Rogers BHG (1976): Complications associated with esophagogastroduodenoscopy and with esophageal dilatation. *Gastrointest Endosc* 23:16–19.
3. Monnier P, Hsieh V, Savary M (1985): Endoscopic treatment of esophageal stenosis using Savary-Gilliard bougies: technical innovations. *Acta Endosc* 15:1–5.
4. Kozarek RA (1987): Esophageal dilation and prostheses. *Endosc Rev* 4:9.
5. Dumon JR, Meric B, Sivac MC, et al (1985): A new method of esophageal dilation using Savary-Gilliard bougies. *Gastrointest Endosc* 31:379.
6. Low DE, Kozarek RA (1988): Esophageal endoscopy, dilation and intraesophageal prosthetic devices. In: *The Esophagus: Surgical and Medical Management*, edited by LD Hill, RA Kozarek, RW McCallum, CD Mercer, p 47. WB Saunders Company, Philadelphia.
7. Kozarek RA (1991): Gastrointestinal dilation. In: *Textbook of Gastroenterology, Vol 2*, p 2. JB Lippincott Company, Philadelphia.

27 / Dilatation of the Esophagus: Pneumatic (Brown-McHardy)

Eugene M. Bozymski

Pneumatic dilatation of the esophagus is one of the major modalities used in the treatment of achalasia. In our department, it is preferred in most instances over surgical myotomy (Heller procedure). The main feature of pneumatic dilatation is that it is a forceful dilatation compared to passive dilatation accomplished by passing a mercury-filled bougie. We use the Brown-McHardy dilator, which consists of a cloth bag of fixed diameter covered by a rubber sheath near the end of a mercury-filled bougie. Air is pumped into this bag and the pressure [pounds per square inch (psi)] monitored on a manometer (Fig. 1). The intended purpose of this forceful dilatation is to decrease the resistance at the lower esophageal sphincter and to allow the esophagus to empty more readily.

A variety of other dilators are available for use in treating the patient with achalasia. These include those that can be attached to an endoscope or passed directly over a flexible guide wire. The latter may be very useful in the patient with a dilated "sigmoid" esophagus.

Indications

1. Achalasia.
2. Certain patients with vigorous achalasia or diffuse esophageal spasm with hypertensive sphincter.

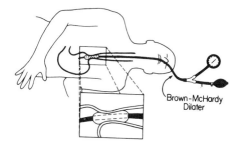

FIG. 1. The pneumatic dilator in place at the lower esophageal sphincter (monitored fluoroscopically).

Contraindications

Absolute

1. Significant bleeding dyscrasia.
2. Esophageal varices.
3. No prior endoscopy.
4. Epiphrenic diverticulum.
5. Recent esophageal mucosal biopsy in the sphincteric area.
6. No prior manometry.

Relative (Depends on the Clinical Situation)

1. Esophagitis (stasis).

Preparation

1. Obtain informed, written consent.
2. Spray the pharynx with a topical anesthetic.
3. Start an intravenous (i.v.) line for administration of atropine and midazolam.

Equipment

1. Endoscope.
2. Gastric lavage tube.

3. Brown-McHardy dilator.
4. Fluoroscope.
5. Gloves and lubricant.

Procedure

1. If there is any debris in the esophagus, empty it with a large-bore gastric lavage tube.
2. Perform upper endoscopy to exclude lesions, such as carcinoma of the fundus presenting as "secondary achalasia" and other diseases of the distal esophagus.
3. Instruct the patient to report with a hand signal when severe chest pain occurs during the dilatation.
4. Pass the Brown-McHardy dilator as one would pass a large, mercury-filled bougie.
5. Position the dilator so that the bag straddles the high-pressure zone. Confirm this fluoroscopically. If positioned too low, the bag is propelled into the stomach with insufflation. If positioned too high, it will retract into the esophagus. When the bag is positioned properly, an hourglass effect is observed (Fig. 2a).
6. Insufflate the bag under fluoroscopic control while the assistant monitors the pressure on the manometer. We have adopted a conservative policy for pneumatic dilatation and would prefer having the patient come back for another dilatation rather than performing the initial procedure too vigorously. In our institution, we use fluoroscopic control and patient response to determine how long to leave the bag inflated. In general, most dilatations require pressures of 9 to 12 psi for 5 to 10 sec to be effective; however, the fluoroscopic appearance and the presence of pain should be guidelines for the extent of dilatation rather than any absolute time or pressure. There are many different methods of forceful dilatation, and it is not known whether the diameter of the bag, the filling pressure of the bag, or the duration of the dilatation is most important in obtaining a good result.
7. Ideally, one of the sides of the hourglass should straighten (Fig. 2b).
8. When the bag straightens or the patient develops severe pain,

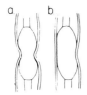

FIG. 2. a: Note the hourglass appearance of the balloon in the lower esophageal sphincter. **b:** The balloon has now expanded on one side.

rapidly deflate the bag and remove the dilator. Most often, small amounts of blood will be noted on the dilating bag following dilatation.

Postprocedure

1. Observe the patient in the hospital overnight following dilatation.
2. Instruct the patient to inform you of continuing chest pain, *back pain*, or pain elsewhere.
3. Monitor vital signs.
4. Elevate the head of the bed.
5. A diatrizoate meglumine (Gastrografin) swallow may be obtained the following morning to study esophageal emptying; however, some physicians recommend an immediate post-dilatation esophagogram to exclude an esophageal perforation.
6. Obtain hematocrit the following morning.
7. Clear liquids for 24 hr and, if clinically stable, soft diet for 2 days, then regular diet.
8. Antacids 30 cc 1 hr p.c. and h.s. for 5 days. Sucralfate slurry has been used in a similar fashion.

Complications

Esophageal Perforation

The dreaded complication of any esophageal dilatation is esophageal perforation (0.6–2.5%) (1,2). This complication should be highly suspect if chest pain persists for more than 15 min following the dilatation or if pain radiates to the back or the left side. The onset of fever is another ominous feature.

Should perforation be suspected, the patient should be taken to the radiology department and a chest X-ray obtained, which may show a left pleural effusion or mediastinal air. Even if normal, the patient should have a Gastrografin swallow to check for a leak. If none is found, barium should then be substituted and the exam repeated. It is important to turn the patient in all positions so that if a leak is present, it will be detected. Once a leak is demonstrated, thoracic surgical consultation should be sought, and most often, surgery is indicated if the leak is discovered early. Others have reported the effective use of antibiotics and parenteral feeding, along with drainage of pleural effusions until the tear closes.

Other Complications

1. Hemorrhage, < 1% to 2%.
2. Aspiration.

REFERENCES

1. Csendes A, Braghetto I, Henriquez A, Cortes C (1989): Late results of prospective randomized study comparing forceful dilatation and esophagomyotomy in patients with achalasia of the esophagus. *Gut* 30:299–304.
2. Vantrappen G, Hellemans J (1980): Treatment of achalasia and related motility disorders. *Gastroenterology* 79:144–154.
3. Rosenow EC (1974): Techniques of esophageal dilatation. In: *The Esophagus*, edited by WS Payne, AM Olsen, pp 55–64. Lea and Febiger, Philadelphia.
4. Jacobs JB, Cohen NL, Mattel S (1983): Pneumatic dilatation as the primary treatment for achalasia. *Ann Otol Rhinol Laryngol* 92:353–356.
5. Witzel L (1981): Treatment of achalasia with a pneumatic dilator attached to a gastroscope. *Endoscopy* 13:176–177.
6. Richter JE (1991): Motility disorders of the esophagus. In: *Textbook of Gastroenterology, Vol 1*, p 1. JB Lippincott Company, Philadelphia.
7. Bozymski EM (1990): Management of esophageal problems. In: *Operative Challenges in Otolaryngology and Head and Neck Surgery*, edited by HC Pillsbury, MM Goldsmith, pp 783–799. Year Book Medical Publishers, Chicago.

28 / Balloon Dilatation of Strictures

William D. Heizer

Most esophageal strictures should be dilated with mercury-filled rubber bougies or wire-guided hard plastic (Savary) dilators. Use of low-compliance hydrostatic balloons for dilatation of strictures in the gastrointestinal tract is a relatively recent innovation. As balloons apply only radial pressure to the narrowed area, it has been assumed that they are safer than traditional methods that involve longitudinal (shearing) forces as well (1–4). However, the reported studies have not confirmed increased safety (3,5). In our opinion, the balloons that have been available until recently are not as effective as the mercury-filled bougies or Savary dilators [see Bozymski's two chapters, "Dilatation of the Esophagus: Mercury-Filled Bougies (Hurst-Maloney)" and "Dilatation of the Esophagus: Wire-Guided Bougies (Eder-Puestow and Savary-Gilliard)"] (3). Recently available balloon dilators that can withstand a higher pressure may prove to be more effective (Bard "no grow" PET balloons, C.R. Bard, Inc., P.O. Box 5069, Billerica, Massachusetts).

Hydrostatic balloon dilatation is especially useful for the initial treatment of upper gastrointestinal strictures that are too narrow or complex for treatment with mercury-filled or Savary dilators (3,4); for through-the-scope (TTS) dilatation of strictures that prevent completion of an endoscopic examination; and for treatment of strictures in the stomach, duodenum, colon, biliary tract, and pancreatic duct that cannot be treated by the older methods (6–10).

Balloon dilators can be positioned across a stricture endoscopically (through the scope) or fluoroscopically. When performed fluoroscopically, the balloon dilator is inserted over a wire that has been placed by endoscopy or fluoroscopy. Placing the dilator without direct visualization or wire guidance is not recommended. Some physicians recommend that all balloon dilatation be done with fluoroscopic observation but we do not use fluoroscopy when performing TTS dilatation. Properly operated, a hydrostatic (water-filled), low-compliance balloon has advantages over a pneumatic (air-filled) balloon. The hydrostatic balloon will not explode forcefully and the pressure will fall rapidly as a stricture begins to dilate or tear, thereby limiting the risk of perforation. Failure to remove most of the air from the water-filled balloon may reduce these advantages.

Many of the technical aspects of hydrostatic balloon dilatation are not established. Consequently, details such as initial balloon size, number of balloon sizes for each dilatation, pressure, and duration of pressure are largely matters of personal choice. The perception that balloons are a relatively inefficient means of stretching and therefore unlikely to cause perforation has led many physicians to use only one relatively large-diameter balloon (4–6 mm larger than the diameter of the stricture) for each dilatation. This technique is most appropriate for dilatation under fluoroscopy where changes in the shape of the balloon can be observed, but is also frequently used for TTS dilatation without fluoroscopy. It is possible that dilatation in one step with a single large balloon is more risky when using the recently available high-pressure balloon dilators. To decrease the possible risk, we and many other users increase the pressure in these balloons in steps, e.g., 5 psi, followed by one-half maximal, three-fourths maximal, and maximal rated pressure. The relative safety of these methods compared to the traditional practice of using three successive balloon dilators of gradually increasing diameter has not been determined.

Indication

1. Dilatation of benign or malignant strictures of the gastrointestinal tract.

Contraindications

Absolute Contraindications

1. Uncooperative patient.
2. Perforation, deep ulcer, or severe inflammation at or near the stricture site.

Relative Contraindications

1. Uncorrectable coagulation disorder.
2. We avoid dilatation for 7 to 10 days following a mucosal biopsy usually by dilating before the biopsy is taken.

Preparation

1. Patient's stomach should be empty.
2. Obtain informed consent.
3. Test the balloon with air for leaks or defects.
4. If fluoroscopic monitoring is used, fill a syringe with 1 part water-soluble contrast solution and 3 parts water. Be sure that the volume of dilute contrast is sufficient to distend fully the largest balloon that will be used.
5. Anesthetize the pharynx with topical anesthesia.
6. Provide intravenous sedation as required.

Equipment

1. Balloon dilators: TTS dilators (Fig. 1a) up to 54 French can pass through the 2.8-mm endoscope channel. For over-the-wire dilatation, balloon dilators are available in sizes from 6 mm in diameter (19 French) to 19 mm in diameter (60 French) (Fig. 1b).
2. Flexible wire guide of appropriate diameter and length.
3. Endoscope and/or fluoroscope, depending on the method to be used.
4. Equipment for mouth suction.

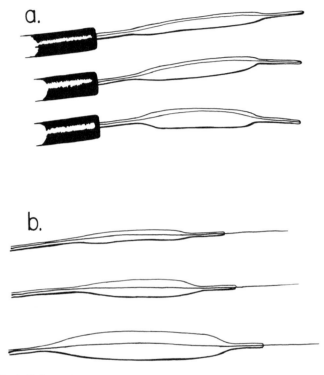

FIG. 1. Balloon dilators. **a:** Through-the-scope (TTS) type. **b:** Over-the-wire type.

Procedure for Hydrostatic Balloon Dilatation Through the Scope

Three-Step Method

1. When the stricture is encountered endoscopically, select a balloon judged to be 2 to 3 mm in diameter larger than the stricture. The balloon should have been tested for leaks, filled with water, and then emptied in such a way that all of the air and as much water as possible has been removed.
2. Apply silicone lubricant to the tip of the catheter and the biopsy channel.
3. Pass the catheter through the stricture under direct vision, attempting to position the middle of the balloon at the middle of the stricture.

4. While observing the pressure gauge, gradually inflate the balloon to its maximum rate pressure with water using the hand-operated pump or syringe supplied by the manufacturer. Take care to avoid exceeding the maximum pressure for the balloon size being used.
5. If the balloon forcibly moves in the direction of its longitudinal axis during inflation, partially deflate it and reposition it in the center of the stricture.
6. Maintain maximum pressure for 30 to 60 sec. If the patient has significant pain, deflate the balloon immediately.
7. Deflate the balloon and observe the stricture. If there is no evidence of significant tear, bleeding, or other damage, repeat steps 1 through 7 using a balloon 2 to 3 mm larger in diameter. Up to three successively larger balloons may be used for each dilatation, if required.

One-Step Method

1. Select a balloon judged to be 6 to 9 mm in diameter larger than the stricture. Balloons 10, 15, or 18 mm in diameter are usually used.
2,3. Same as above.
4. Inflate the balloon to 5 psi and maintain that pressure 30 to 60 sec. If tolerated with no more than mild pain, increase pressure successively to one-half, three-fourths, and full maximum rated pressure, maintaining each pressure for 30 to 60 sec.
5,6. Same as above.

These techniques are suitable for dilatation of any stricture in the upper gastrointestinal tract that the upper endoscope can reach. For pyloric strictures, special balloons, shorter than those used for the esophagus, are used so that the tip will not damage the duodenal bulb.

Procedure for Hydrostatic Balloon Dilatation over a Wire

1. Under endoscopic or fluoroscopic control, pass the balloon dilator wire across the stricture until the flexible tip of the wire lies at least 15 to 20 cm distal to the stricture.

2. Choose a balloon dilator based on the one-step or three-step procedure described for TTS dilatation.
3. Pass the deflated balloon over the wire until the radiopaque markers at each end of the balloon straddle the estimated location of the stricture. If endoscopy has been done, use the incisor-to-stricture measurement to mark the balloon dilator shaft so that when the mark is at the incisors, the balloon will straddle the stricture. It is preferable to position the balloon 2 to 3 cm too distal than too proximal.
4. Slowly instill diluted contrast material into the balloon and, if needed, withdraw the loosely filled balloon until it straddles the stricture, as indicated by a waist in the midportion of the balloon (Fig. 2A).
5. Inflate the balloon to maximum pressure either gradually or stepwise and maintain the pressure for 30 to 60 sec or less depending on patient discomfort and appearance of the balloon under fluoroscopy.
6. Observe the balloon with short bursts of fluoroscopy to note the increase in diameter of the stricture (i.e., loss of the waist, Fig. 2B). The amount and duration of pressure should be determined by the appearance of the waist, patient discomfort, and previous experience with the particular stricture.

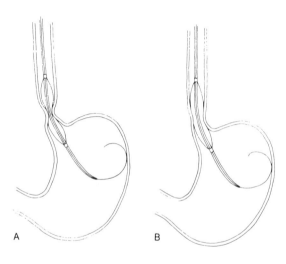

A   B   **FIG. 2.**

Postprocedure

1. Instruct the patient not to eat or drink anything until the topical anesthetic has worn off.
2. Liquid diet for 4 hr.
3. Instruct the patient what to do if gastrointestinal bleeding or severe chest pain or abdominal pain should occur.
4. Review and reinstruct the patient regarding antireflux treatment if the stricture is acid peptic in origin.

Complications

The true incidence of complications is unknown. A retrospective survey reported in 1986 (5) uncovered 11 hemorrhages and 2 perforations in 617 balloon dilatations of the esophagus, 4 perforations and 1 hemorrhage among 545 gastric dilatations, and 3 perforations and 2 hemorrhages following 64 colon dilatations. Many of these complications were attributed to the sharp tip of the early balloon dilators. Other potential complications include aspiration, allergic reactions, and bacteremia. Cholangitis and pancreatitis appear to occur with rather high frequency following balloon dilatations of biliary and pancreatic duct strictures (5).

REFERENCES

1. Graham DY (1985): Dilatation for the management of benign and malignant strictures of the esophagus. In: *Therapeutic Gastrointestinal Endoscopy*, edited by SE Silvis, pp 1–30. Igaku-Shoin, New York.
2. Starck E, Paolucci V, Herzer M, Crummy AB (1984): Esophageal stenosis: treatment with balloon catheters. *Radiology* 95:637–640.
3. Shemesh E, Czerniak A (1990): Comparison between Savary-Gilliard and balloon dilatation of benign esophageal strictures. *World J Surg* 14: 518–522.
4. Graham DY, Tabibian N, Schwartz JT, Smith JL (1987): Evaluation of the effectiveness of through-the-scope balloons as dilators of benign and malignant gastrointestinal strictures. *Gastrointest Endosc* 33:432–435.
5. Kozarek RA (1986): Hydrostatic balloon dilatation of gastrointestinal stenoses: a national survey. *Gastrointest Endosc* 32:15–18.
6. Dinneen MD, Moston RW (1991): Treatment of colonic anastomotic strictures with 'through the scope' balloon dilators. *J R Soc Med* 84: 264–266.

7. Banerjee AK, Walters TK, Wilkins R, Burke M (1991): Wire-guided balloon coloplasty—a new treatment for colorectal strictures? *J R Soc Med* 84:136–139.

8. Williams AJK, Palmer KR (1991): Endoscopic balloon dilatation as a therapeutic option in the management of intestinal strictures resulting from Crohn's disease. *Br J Surg* 78:453–454.

9. Fregonese D, Di Falco G, Di Toma F (1990): Balloon dilatation of anastomotic intestinal stenoses: long-term results. *Endoscopy* 22:249–253.

10. Sataloff DM, Lieber CP, Seinige UL. (1990): Strictures following gastric stapling for morbid obesity: results of endoscopic dilatation. *Am Surg* 56:167–174.

29 / Ablation of Bleeding (Nonvariceal) Gastrointestinal Lesions

Douglas A. Drossman

The methods commonly used for ablating nonvariceal bleeding gastrointestinal lesions (ulcer vessels, angiodysplasia, Mallory-Weiss tears) involve monopolar and bipolar/multipolar coagulation,[1] heater probe treatment, and injection of vasoconstrictive or sclerosing agents. Laser therapy (see chapter by Isaacs et al, "Laser Therapy of Gastrointestinal Disease") is a more expensive and less available technique that does not afford the same degree of portability. The injecting devices easily pass through the endoscope biopsy channel, and treatment is effective in stopping acute bleeding episodes up to 90% of the time. Effectiveness decreases when: (a) the bleeding is from a large-caliber (serosal) vessel, (b) the lesion is relatively inaccessible (e.g., postbulbar), (c) a coagulation disorder is present, or (d) repeated treatments are needed.

Monopolar Electrocoagulation (1)

This involves generation of high-frequency electrical energy from the probe through the tissue to a distal electrode at a site on the patient's body. The electrical energy, activated by a foot pedal, generates heat to coagulate the vessel. Monopolar coagulation was the first effective ablative technique to be developed. It is now less frequently used because *en face* contact is usually needed for effective hemostasis, and the depth of injury is difficult to regulate.

---

[1]Coagulation produces tissue necrosis without cutting by either fulguration (sparking of tissue) or dessication (no sparking—direct contact).

Bipolar/Multipolar Electrocoagulation (2)

With this method, the potential for deep tissue injury is reduced, since the electrodes are limited to the area of the probe; however, a larger number of applications are usually needed to stop the bleeding. The most popular bipolar electrode system is the BICAP (Microvasive, Watertown, Massachusetts). The device contains a circumferentially placed, six-bipolar electrode oriented around a cylinder 7 mm in length. It is available in 7 French and 10 French diameter sizes, and is also attached to a water pump.

Heater Probe (3)

Direct heat thermal cautery transfers energy to tissue by thermal conduction. The energy produced by a miniaturized heating coil is regulated by a thermometer in the tip that feeds back to the computerized power source. Energy transfer occurs in a controlled fashion, and at a relatively low temperature (250°), thereby limiting the degree of tissue injury. We use the Heat Probe unit (Olympus Company, Lake Success, New York) (available in 2.4 and 3.2 mm sizes) almost exclusively for coagulation because:

1. The depth of injury is limited to 1 to 3 mm.
2. There is little electrical hazard to the patient.
3. Coagulation can be performed tangentially.
4. The device is portable and inexpensive.
5. Water flow and energy settings may be preset.
6. Washing and tamponade can be done simultaneously.
7. Tissue adherence is minimized through use of the Teflon coating.

Injection Therapy (4,5)

Injection therapy is the most recent ablative technique for the control of nonvariceal hemorrhage. It appears to be as effective as electrocoagulation (6) and heater probe treatment (7) and is less expensive. The injector (Microvasive, Watertown, Massachusetts) is also used for variceal sclerotherapy. It consists of a disposable, small-diameter (2-mm) catheter with a No. 25 gauge needle at the tip that can extend 5 mm from its retracted position. Any of a variety of liquid agents (dilute epinephrine, morrhuate sodium, absolute ethanol) can be used. An injection initially causes volume-dependent cessation of bleeding by pressure effect and, depending on the agent, can also produce vasoconstriction, acute inflammation, clot formation, and scarring. We find that injection therapy is particularly useful during active bleeding when precise placement of a probe is difficult. We use dilute epinephrine as the sole form of initial treatment, or to slow the bleeding prior to heater probe treatment. Adverse cardiac effects may potentially occur from systemic absorption of epinephrine. However, to our knowledge, none have yet been reported.

Indications

1. To stop bleeding from gastrointestinal lesions:
   a. Ulcers.
   b. Arteriovenous malformations (angiodysplasia).
   c. Localized gastritis.
   d. Mallory-Weiss tears.
   e. Postpolypectomy or -sphincterotomy complications.
2. To prevent bleeding from lesions at high risk to bleed:
   a. Visible vessels, sentinel clot, marginal oozing, red spot (in decreasing order of risk) on an ulcer.
   b. Arteriovenous malformations.

Contraindications

1. Uncooperative patient.
2. Massively bleeding lesion.
3. Inability to place the probe or injector properly.
4. Bleeding from esophageal varices (unless a variceal sclerosant is used; see chapter by Bozymski, "Endoscopic Sclerosis of Esophageal Varices").
5. Evidence for perforation at bleeding site.
6. Arteriovenous malformations larger than 1 cm may be difficult to ablate because of large submucosal feeding vessels.

Equipment

1. Large-channel (preferably double-channel) endoscope and accessory equipment (see chapters by Sartor, "Upper Gastrointestinal Endoscopy," and Drossman, "Colonoscopy").
2. Large-bore Edlich tube for gastric irrigation prior to treatment.
3. Coagulation or heater probe setup with transformer units.
4. Sclerotherapy needle with epinephrine or sclerosant.
5. Crash cart with cardiac monitoring unit.

Preparation

1. Pretest all electrical equipment to ensure that it is in proper working order. Attach the distant electrode for monopolar coagulation.
2. Be certain that the patient is clinically stable and is being continually monitored.
3. Remove blood and clots using an Edlich tube if there is gastroduodenal bleeding and, if possible, administer an oral lavage prep (e.g., GoLYTELY, Colyte) for colonic bleeding.

Procedure

1. Perform an emergency upper endoscopy (see Sartor's chapter, "Emergency Upper Gastrointestinal Endoscopy") or colonoscopy (see Drossman's chapter, "Colonoscopy") to confirm the site of bleeding and to identify other gastrointestinal lesions.
2. Decide which lesions will be treated. In our unit, we coagulate all actively bleeding lesions and usually coagulate certain high-risk nonbleeding lesions (e.g., fresh clot on lesion, visible vessel). For multiple lesions (e.g., angiodysplasia), treat the most dependent lesions first to maintain visibility of all lesions if bleeding occurs.
3. Set the energy level for the coagulator or heater probe based on the manufacturer's recommendations and previous experience with the technique.
4. Wash away any blood or clot from any area to be coagulated.

Do not apply energy pulses through blood, since this produces a coagulum that will raise tissue impedence. If blood is seen oozing from a clot in the base of an ulcer, gently dislodge and lift away the clot with the probe tip or other device. This technique is not usually necessary for injection therapy if the lesion is well seen.

5. *Heater probe treatment* (Fig. 1):
   a. Apply firm pressure *en face* sufficient to tamponade (coapt) an actively bleeding lesion. If the vessel is not bleeding, it may be preferable to first apply several treatments around the vessel, thereby minimizing the risk of inducing bleeding.
   b. Give up to several heater probe pulses while holding position to coapt or seal the walls of the vessel.
      i. Large arteries—three to six 20-J pulses.
      ii. Angiodysplasia—one to three 5- to 10-J pulses. Larger lesions (> 7 mm in diameter) may first require circumferential applications beginning at the periphery. Avoid overdistension of the bowel.
      iii. Mallory-Weiss tear—two to three 20-J pulses. These lesions almost always require tangential placement of the probe.
   c. Press the wash button briefly to dislodge the tip before manually lifting the probe from the lesion.

6. *Bipolar coagulation*:
   a. If possible, use a larger (3.2-mm) probe because it provides better tamponade, washing is more efficient, and the coagulation zone is greater, thereby achieving better hemostasis.
   b. Tamponade an arterial vessel and coagulate with 5- to 10-sec pulses with a power setting determined from prior experience with the transformer. Some endoscopists prefer to coagulate circumferentially around a bleeding lesion before applying coagulation directly. With the newer, stiffer probe tips, tangential applications can also be done.
   c. For treating colonic angiodysplastic bleeding, use a lower power setting, avoid overdistension of the bowel, and do not tamponade.

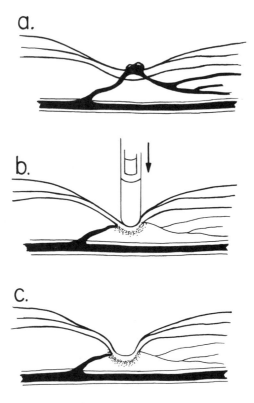

FIG. 1. Heater probe treatment. **a:** Visible vessel seen above the surface of the ulcer crature. **b:** Heat applied by the probe that is tamponading the vessel. **c:** Postprocedure view showing the sealed vessel.

7. *Injection therapy:*
   a. Inject the agent at three or four sites surrounding the bleeding lesion to raise an edema cuff and compress the bleeding vessel.
   b. If the lesion is too tangential for direct treatment, an injection behind the bleeding site may bring it into better position.
   c. The injection volume depends on the type of agent. We use up to 10 ml of 1:10,000 epinephrine diluted in saline. To avoid unneeded tissue necrosis, injection therapy should be discontinued as soon as the bleeding stops.

Complications

1. Continued or induced bleeding.
2. Ulceration.
3. Perforation.

The success and complication rates are more dependent on the skill of the endoscopist than the specific method (8).

REFERENCES

1. Papp JP (1982): Endoscopic electrocoagulation in the management of upper gastrointestinal tract bleeding. *Surg Clin North Am* 62:797–806.
2. Laine L (1987): Multipolar electrocoagulation in the treatment of active upper gastrointestinal tract hemmorrhage. *N Engl J Med* 316:1613–1617.
3. Storey DW (1983): Endoscopic control of peptic ulcer hemorrhage using the "Heater Probe." *Gut* 24:967–970.
4. Panes J, Forne M, Marco C, et al (1987): Controlled trial of endoscopic sclerosis in bleeding peptic ulcers. *Lancet* 2:1291–1294.
5. Chung SCS, Leung JWC, Steele RJC, et al (1988): Endoscopic injection of adrenaline for actively bleeding ulcers: a randomized trial. *Br Med J* 296:1631–1633.
6. Waring JP, Sanowski RA, Sawyer RL, et al (1991): A randomized comparison of multipolar electrocoagulation and injection sclerosis for the treatment of peptic ulcer. *Gastrointest Endosc* 37:295–298.
7. Chung SCS, Leung JWC, Sung JY, et al (1991): Injection or heat probe for bleeding ulcer. *Gastroenterology* 100:33–37.
8. Jensen DM (1991): Endoscopic control of nonvariceal upper gastrointestinal hemorrhage. In: *Textbook of Gastroenterology*, edited by T Yamada, DH Alpers, C Owyang, DW Powell, FE Silverstein, pp 2618–2634. JB Lippincott Company, Philadelphia.

30 / Laser Therapy of Gastrointestinal Disease

Kim L. Isaacs, Donald P. Brannan, and
Eugene M. Bozymski

During the 1980s there was tremendous growth in the technology and application of lasers in gastroenterology for hemostasis, tumor ablation, and lithotripsy (biliary stones). The most commonly used laser in the therapy of gastrointestinal disease in the 1990s is the neodynium yttrium-aluminum-garnet (Nd:YAG) laser. Pulsed infrared lasers and tunable dye lasers with an adjustable output are also being utilized in selected clinical situations. Infrared lasers have a high tissue absorbance and are used for tissue ablation, whereas tunable dye lasers have a variable wavelength output and are used for laser lithotripsy as well as tumor ablation (1).

Currently the use of lasers in gastroenterology depends on their function as thermal devices. The heat delivered vaporizes tissue for tumor ablation and coagulates tissue for hemostasis. With most commercial Nd:YAG lasers, power outputs up to 100 W can be selected. When the temperature of the tissue is raised to 60°C, coagulation occurs. At temperatures of 100°C, vaporization will occur (2). Tissue temperature is determined by the wattage output and the duration of the laser pulse. By using high outputs (i.e., 80–100 W) and longer pulse durations (i.e., >0.5 sec) at close distances, tissue vaporization occurs. Additionally, contact probes are also available.

In this chapter we will concentrate on the use of the Nd:YAG laser in the treatment of chronic hemorrhage and in the treatment of esophageal malignancies.

Indications

1. Coagulation
   a. Acute hemorrhage: active bleeding, visible vessel[1].
   b. Chronic hemorrhage: angiodysplasia, hemorrhoids, radiation changes (3) (colitis/proctitis), antral vascular ectasia ("watermelon stomach") (4).
2. Tumor ablation
   a. Esophageal malignancy: squamous cell or adenocarcinoma (2,5,6).
   b. Rectal carcinoma: in conjunction with radiation therapy.
   c. Selected benign or malignant lesions of the gastrointestinal tract (7).

Contraindications

Absolute

1. Any condition that would preclude safe endoscopy (see chapter by Sartor, "Upper Gastrointestinal Endoscopy").
2. Inability to adequately visualize area to be treated.
3. Inspired oxygen levels greater than 50%.

Relative

1. Myocardial ischemia.
2. Severe pulmonary disease (intubation may be required to proceed safely).
3. Coagulopathy.
4. Recent administration of photosensitive compounds.
5. Esophageal-tracheal fistula.

---

[1]Other modalities such as heater probe or BICAP [see Drossman's chapter, "Ablation of Bleeding (Nonvariceal) Gastrointestinal Lesions"] are as effective, more portable, and less expensive (1).

Preparation

1. Obtain informed consent, explaining risks and benefits of laser therapy and other potential treatment modalities.
2. Prepare patient for appropriate endoscopic procedure: upper GI tract (upper endoscopy: see Sartor's chapter "Upper Gastrointestinal Endoscopy"), lower GI tract (colonoscopy preparation: see Drossman's chapter "Colonscopy").
3. Place protective ophthalmic safety glasses on patient.
4. Sedate patient as appropriate. Most patients will tolerate procedure with conscious intravenous (i.v.) sedation (e.g., meperidine and midolazam, see Isaacs' chapter "Medications in the Gastrointestinal Procedure Unit"). Selected patients (e.g., large tumor burden, respiratory difficulties) may require general anesthesia.
5. Antibiotic prophylaxis in patients with valvular heart disease. (See Isaacs' chapter, "Medications in the Gastrointestinal Procedure Unit").

Selected Equipment

1. Nd:YAG laser unit. Several are commercially available.
2. Assortment of laser fibers (sheathed or unsheathed, contact or noncontact).
3. Room with special electrical power, adequate water supply, and drain capacity for laser. Some of the newer air-cooled lasers may require no room adaptation.
4. Video endoscopy equipment is preferred to allow observation by the surgical team and support staff.
5. The endoscope should be equipped with a white ceramic tip to prevent heat damage to the endoscope tip.
6. Ophthalmic safety equipment for all personnel.

Procedure

General Considerations: Hemostasis

Multiple studies have been performed using laser therapy for the treatment of acutely bleeding lesions such as peptic ulcers and variceal bleeding (1). The use of laser therapy in this clinical situation has been largely replaced by more portable therapeutic intervention such as the heater probe (for PUD) and injection sclerotherapy for esophageal varices [see Drossman's chapter, "Ablation of Bleeding (Nonvariceal) Gastrointestinal Lesions," and Bozymski's chapter, "Endoscopic Sclerosis of Esophageal Varices"] (8). Now lasers are most commonly used for photoablation of numerous vascular malformations responsible for chronic blood loss (see above), although heater probe and multipolar and bipolar electrocoagulation can also be utilized. The procedure will be described using antral vascular ectasia "watermelon stomach" as the prototypic lesion.

General Considerations: Tumor Ablation

Variations in technique exist with respect to (a) use of contact or noncontact probes, or (b) the use of high power (>50 W) or low power (<50 W). A discussion of the pros and cons of these different techniques is beyond the scope of this chapter [see (1) for excellent review of these topics] (5). Either an antegrade or retrograde approach may be used for initial tumor ablation (Fig. 1). Both methods have advantages and disadvantages. The ante-

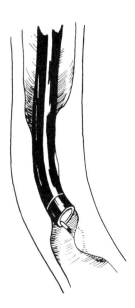

FIG. 1. Retrograde method of esophageal tumor ablation using laser therapy.

grade approach requires multiple treatment sessions. The retrograde approach requires the ability to pass the endoscope beyond the distal margin of the lesion and generally will require pre-procedure dilation. It offers the potential advantage of complete treatment in a single session. We will describe a "standard technique" utilizing a retrograde noncontact approach. A combination retrograde and antegrade approach may be necessary in some patients (5). No absolute energy maximum need be set for a treatment session. A rough correlation exists between the tumor length (volume) and the energy requirements for tumor destruction (6).

Procedure

1. Prepare the laser unit per manufacturer's instructions.
2. Place the unit on standby.
3. Perform endoscopy in standard fashion to identify landmarks and the lesion(s) to be treated.
4. The bare laser fiber may be placed into a plastic sheath or into medical-grade tubing to protect the endoscope from the sharp tip of the laser fiber and for easier manipulation.
5. Insert the sheathed laser fiber into the biopsy port of the endoscope and pass the fiber sheath unit until it is visible at the end of the endoscope. Pull back the sheath to expose the laser fiber. The aiming beams may be used to focus on the tissue. *Do not activate the laser fiber within the endoscope. The endoscope will be damaged by the thermal energy produced by the laser.*
6. Put on protective eye gear.
7. Activate the laser and treat the lesion.
8. Treatment of arteriovenous malformations:
   a. Identify the lesion to be treated and place the endoscope tip at the distal margin of the lesion.
   b. Begin with a power setting less than 30 W and a pulse duration of less than 0.2 sec. The range of power used is 10 to 70 W. Increase the wattage to obtain adequate photocoagulation as manifested by a white coagulum at the treatment site. Pulse duration ranges from 0.1 to 0.5 sec.
   c. Multiple sessions may be required to photocoagulate all

lesions. Tissue edema may prevent coagulation of all lesions during a single setting. Retreatment is performed at 2- to 3-month intervals (2).

9. Ablation of esophageal carcinoma:
   a. Identify the location and geometry of the esophageal lesion.
   b. If unable to pass the endoscope beyond the distal margin of the tumor, pass a guide wire under direct visualization and perform a dilatation [usually with wire-guided dilators, see Bozymski's chapter, "Dilatation of the Esophagus: Wire-Guided Bougies (Eder-Puestow and Savary-Gilliard)"] under fluoroscopic guidance to obtain a lumen diameter of approximately 15 mm.
   c. Position the endoscope at the distal margin of the tumor (Fig. 1).
   d. Treat the lesion with the Nd:YAG laser set at 40 to 70 W (0.5–1-sec pulse duration) starting at the distal margin and treating more proximally as the endoscope is withdrawn. Higher power settings lead to tissue vaporization, which increases the risk of perforation and bleeding (9).
   e. Debridement and irrigation are carried out as needed throughout the procedure.
   f. Avoid excessive air insufflation and aspirate air as necessary.
   g. The decision to retreat the lesion is dependent on the functional result, i.e., ability to eat. Lesions may be retreated as early as 48 to 72 hr after the first treatment (5).

Postprocedure

1. Remove protective eye gear after laser has been deactivated.
2. Assure stability of patient prior to transfer to recovery area.
3. The postprocedure note should include:
   a. Exam findings.
   b. Extent of lesion treated.
   c. Total number of joules used for session.
   d. Sedation used.
   e. Complications.
4. Clean endoscopic and laser equipment.

Complications (Esophageal Tumor Ablation)

Major (5%)

1. Esophageal perforation, 2.1%.
2. Fistula formation, 0.8%.
3. Severe hemorrhage, 0.7%.
4. Sepsis, 0.6%.

Minor

1. Worsening of obstruction 24–48 hours later, due to edema.
2. Transient bacteremia.
3. Vagal reactions.
4. Mild chest pain.
5. Leukocytosis.

Efficacy

No controlled trials have been performed to determine overall efficacy of laser photocoagulation for vascular malformations. Case series suggest an improvement in chronic gastrointestinal blood loss of up to 90% (4).

For esophageal tumor ablation, success of lumen recanalization is achieved in about 90% to 95% of those treated. Functional success, defined as the restored ability to eat solids when only liquids were able to be taken previously, is achieved in 70% to 80%.

REFERENCES

1. Deschner W, Fleischer D (1991): GI laser therapy: what's in store? *Contemp Gastroenterol* 4:8–22.
2. Fleischer D, Kessler F (1983): Endoscopic Nd-YAG laser therapy for carcinoma of the esophagus: a new form of palliative treatment. *Gastroenterology* 85:600–606.
3. Alexander T, Dwyer R (1988): Endoscopic Nd:YAG laser treatment of severe radiation injury of the lower gastrointestinal tract: long term follow-up. *Gastrointest Endosc* 34:407–411.
4. Gostout C, Ahlquist D, Viggiano T, et al (1989): Endoscopic laser therapy for watermelon stomach. *Gastroenterology* 96:1462–1465.

5. Fleischer D (1989): Endoscopic laser therapy for esophageal cancer: emphasis on past and future. *Lasers Surg Med* 9:6–16.
6. Pietrafitta J (1987): Endoscopic laser therapy for the treatment of malignant esophageal obstruction. *Lasers Surg Med* 7:487–490.
7. Eckhauser M (1987): Endoscopic laser vaporization of obstructing left colonic cancer to avoid decompressive colostomy. *Gastrointest Endosc* 33:105–106.
8. (1989): NIH Consensus Development Conference on therapeutic endoscopy and bleeding ulcers. *JAMA* 262:1369–1372.
9. Hunter J (1989): Endoscopic laser applications and the gastrointestinal tract. *Surg Clin North Am* 69:1147–1165.

31 / Endoscopic Sclerosis of Esophageal Varices

Eugene M. Bozymski

Bleeding from esophageal varices is one of the most difficult problems confronting gastroenterologists and surgeons. A wide variety of therapeutic maneuvers have been developed to control the bleeding. Currently, one way to control hemorrhage on a long-term basis is the use of decompressive portal systemic shunt surgery; however, many patients, because of coexisting medical problems (usually decompensated liver disease) or because of technical problems, are not suitable shunt candidates. It is this group of patients that led Terblanche to reintroduce endoscopic sclerosis of varices, which had been practiced many years earlier. Sclerotherapy has been shown to be effective in controlling bleeding in the acute situation and also is effective in the long-term management of this type of patient. The vascular radiologist may contribute to the management of such patients by establishing a portosystemic shunt by the use of a self-expanding metallic stent placed via a transjugular approach (TIPSS).

Indications

1. To stop acute hemorrhage from esophageal varices.
2. To ablate esophageal varices causing recurrent hemorrhage.
3. Temporizing measure to control bleeding in patients with poor hepatic reserve in anticipation of shunt surgery, or liver transplantation if the condition warrants.
4. Patients with variceal hemorrhage who are not operative candidates.

Contraindications

1. Uncooperative patient.
2. More than mildly abnormal clotting factors.

Preparation

1. Patient should have been seen by Vascular Surgery Service.
2. Obtain written, informed consent.
3. Blood sample in blood bank.
4. Establish venous access.
5. Meperidine, midazolam, atropine, and glucagon should be available.

Equipment

1. We use a twin-channel gastroscope and direct puncture of the varix followed by injection.
2. Injector (No. 23 gauge, 4-mm needle). A variety of disposable injectors are also available from a number of suppliers. The injector should be tested for patency prior to use.
3. Two to three 10-cc syringes filled with 5% morrhuate sodium or ethanolamine oleate, 5%.
4. Safety goggles.
5. TV monitor (greatly preferred) or teaching attachment.
6. Gloves and lubricant.

Procedure

1. Anesthetize the patient's pharynx with topical anesthetic.
2. Premedicate the patient with 0.5 mg atropine, along with meperidine and midazolam as needed.
3. Pass the gastroscope.
4. Inspect the esophagus, stomach, and duodenum for other possible sources of bleeding (see Sartor's chapter, "Emergency Upper Gastrointestinal Endoscopy").
5. Identify the esophageal varices and note their extent.
6. The physician and assistants must put protective safety goggles in place and place a towel over the patient's eyes to protect against accidental spraying of sclerosing agent.
7. Reposition the scope to identify the varices just above the esophagogastric junction.
8. Pass the injector until it is visualized in the lumen over the varix and impale it. On command, the assistant injects 1 to 2 cc sclerosant (Fig. 1).

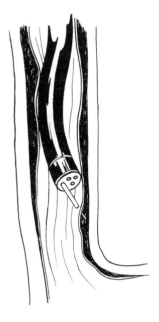

FIG. 1. Sclerotherapy injection. The varix is impaled by the ejected needle to inject sclerosant.

9. Remove the needle and observe the varix for excessive bleeding.
10. Sequentially inject all varices present at a given level. Advance the gastroscope into the stomach and aspirate air.
11. Move the scope cephalad 4 to 5 cm and repeat the procedure.
12. Again withdraw the endoscope approximately 4 cm and repeat the injection.
13. If a specific vein is to be injected at multiple sites, use smaller volumes (0.5–1.5 cc).
14. Remove the air from the stomach and remove the scope.
15. Other helpful hints:
    a. Do not inject greater than a total of approximately 20 cc sclerosing agent during one procedure.
    b. Expect to see either blanching or discoloration of the vein with some injections.
    c. If a bleb begins to form at the injection site, stop—it may be too superficial.

    d. If a bleeding point is identified on a varix, inject the varix below this point. If this is not possible due to excess blood, inject above or to the side of the bleeding point and then below. Some injections intended to be intravariceal will be paravariceal.

    e. Some patients may experience pain at the time of injection.

    f. Intravenous (i.v.) glucagon may be helpful in decreasing esophageal motility.

    g. Some physicians prefer to do paravariceal injections. This technique involves injecting smaller volumes of sclerosant (0.5–1 cc per injection) *between* the varices at the level of the esophagogastric junction. In theory, this technique leads to a fibrous band in the distal esophagus that prevents bleeding but may not obliterate the varices. In practice, some paravariceal injections will be intravariceal and vice versa.

16. Sclerotherapy may be repeated in 4 to 5 days and then again in a few weeks. Further sclerotherapy is then planned as needed.

17. Some endoscopists use balloon tamponade during sclerotherapy. If this is thought necessary, cut the end off a condom and make it into a simple sheath. Place it over the distal part of the endoscope and double it back over itself. Fix it at its distal end by a rubber band. Slide a polyethylene tube into the condom at its proximal end, which is also fixed by rubber bands. Tape the small polyethylene tube along the shaft of the endoscope. Then, attach a syringe to this catheter and blow air into the balloon for inflation purposes. Air can be deflated from the balloon by aspiration. Then, follow these procedures:

    a. When the varix to be injected is chosen, blow up the balloon with approximately 25 cc air.

    b. Inject the varix and deflate the balloon.

    c. If bleeding persists after the injection, advance the scope a few centimeters so that the balloon portion is over the puncture site and inflate the balloon for 4 min. This usually controls the bleeding. If it persists, infuse i.v. vasopressin. Proceed with further injections as needed.

Postprocedure

1. Monitor vital signs.
2. Observe for any further signs of gastrointestinal blood loss.
3. When the patient's normal pharyngeal function has returned, clear liquid diet is permitted and continued for 24 hr.
4. Bed rest until the following morning.
5. Antacid 30 cc every hr while awake for the remainder of the day and then five to six times a day for the next 5 days. A sucralfate slurry can be used—1 g q.i.d.—in a similar fashion.
6. Liquid H_2 receptor antagonist p.o. every 12 hr for the next 5 days.
7. Hematocrit 6 hr post procedure and again the following morning.

Complications

1. Hemorrhage from tearing the varix with the needle.
2. Perforation.
3. Pleural effusion.
4. Ulceration of the esophagus at injection sites.
5. Postprocedure fever.
6. Retrosternal pain may persist for a few days.
7. Esophageal stricture may be a late complication.

BIBLIOGRAPHY

1. Terblanche J (1985): A review of injection sclerotherapy—the Cape Town experience. *Jpn J Surg* 15:103–111.
2. VanHootegem P, Rutgeerts P, Fevery J, Broeckaert L, deGroote J, Vantrappen G (1984): Sclerotherapy of oesophageal varices after variceal hemorrhage. *Endoscopy* 16:95–97.
3. Health and Public Policy Committee, American College of Physicians (1984): Endoscopic sclerotherapy for esophageal varices. *Ann Intern Med* 100:608–610.
4. Sivak MV Jr (1985): Sclerotherapy for esophageal varices. In: *Therapeutic Gastrointestinal Endoscopy*, edited by SE Silvis, pp 31–66. Igaku-Shoin, New York.
5. Fleig WE, Stange EF, Ruettenauer K, Ditschcuneit H (1983): Emergency

endoscopic sclerotherapy for bleeding esophageal varices: a prospective study in patients not responding to balloon tamponade. *Gastrointest Endosc* 29:8–14.

6. The Copenhagen Esophageal Varices Sclerotherapy Project (1984): Sclerotherapy after first variceal hemorrhage in cirrhosis: a randomized multicenter trial. *N Engl J Med* 311:1594–1600.

7. Cello JP, Grendell JH, Crass RA, Trunkey DD, Cobb EE, Heilbron DC (1984): Endoscopic sclerotherapy portacaval shunt in patients with severe cirrhosis and variceal hemorrhage. *N Engl J Med* 311:1589–1594.

8. Paquet KJ (1982): Prophylactic endoscopic sclerosing treatment of the esophageal wall in varices—a prospective controlled randomized trial. *Endoscopy* 14:4–5.

32 / Percutaneous Endoscopic Gastrostomy

Eugene M. Bozymski

There are many patients in whom long-term enteral nutritional support is necessary. Patients with strokes or head and neck tumors that interfere with normal swallowing function previously have required a surgically placed gastrostomy or jejunostomy tube for nutritional support, since placement of a long-term enteral feeding tube via the nasogastric route is not practical. The development of an endoscopic technique for the placement of a gastrostomy tube has been a very useful adjunct in the management of such patients and has become the treatment of choice. In this chapter, the two major techniques of percutaneous endoscopic gastrostomy (PEG) are outlined. There are many self-contained kits that are commercially available and we tend to favor those that feature a gastrostomy tube that can be removed and replaced without requiring additional endoscopy.

Indications

1. To provide an access for nutritional support in patients with an abnormality of the swallowing mechanism or in whom oral intake of food is precluded and long-term placement of an enteral feeding tube is not satisfactory.
2. Patients who demonstrate a potential for response to nutritional support.

Contraindications

1. Ascites.
2. Morbid obesity.

3. Extensive scarring of the anterior abdominal wall.
4. Significant bleeding diathesis.
5. Gastric outlet obstruction.
6. Esophageal obstruction.
7. Airway obstruction that would preclude introduction or removal of the PEG tube.
8. Portal hypertension with portal gastropathy.

Preparation

1. Obtain operative consent from the patient or if necessary from a responsible family member.
2. Nothing by mouth for 12 hr.
3. Place an intravenous line to administer meperidine, midazolam, and atropine.
4. Remove dentures.
5. Administer prophylactic antibiotics, such as ampicillin or a cephalosporin.

Equipment

1. Upper endoscope with video monitor.
2. Topical anesthetic, tongue blades, and emesis basin.
3. Polyp snare.
4. Bite block and lubricant.
5. Gastrostomy-related equipment:
   a. Disposable lap pack.
   b. Prep tray, including razor, alcohol, povidone-iodine (Betadine), and sterile sponge sticks.
   c. No. 11 scalpel.
   d. Masks, gowns, caps, shoe covers, and sterile gloves.
   e. 1% Xylocaine (lidocaine) with syringe and 25 gauge needle.
   f. Commercially available guide wire–type PEG system with soft retention dome (removable without endoscopy) gastrostomy tube.

Procedure 1

1. Place the patient in approximately a 10° to 15° head-up, supine recumbent position. With the patient in this position, the

team must carefully observe for the possibility of aspiration. Frequent suction may be needed.

2. If the patient is not cooperative, arm restraint with a blanket may be needed.

3. Prep the abdomen first using alcohol and then povidone-iodine in circular motions, beginning from the proposed gastrostomy site and working outward. Drape the abdomen with towel drapes and a lap sheet.

4. Perform a standard diagnostic upper endoscopy (see Sartor's chapter, "Upper Gastrointestinal Endoscopy") and identify the site for the gastrostomy tube. This site is located approximately one-third the distance from the left costal margin to the umbilicus. It is chosen by inflating the stomach in a darkened room, transilluminating the abdominal wall in the appropriate chosen area, and then having the assistant push in the anterior abdominal wall so that one can see the finger indenting the anterior wall of the stomach.

5. Pass the snare through the biopsy channel of the scope and position it near the chosen gastrostomy site.

6. Inject several milliliters of Xylocaine into the anterior abdominal wall and make an adequate (> 1 cm) skin incision. Thrust the Seldinger needle in a perpendicular direction through the stab wound and through the anterior wall of the stomach under direct vision. Loop the cannula with the snare.

7. Remove the needle stylet of the cannula and pass the flexible end of the guide wire through the cannula into the stomach.

8. At this point the snare is loosened from the cannula and allowed to slide over the guide wire which is grasped by the snare (Fig. 1a).

9. Retract the endoscope, snare, and guide wire in tandem and pull them through the patient's mouth (Fig. 1b).

10. Remove the cannula from the stomach. At this time, the guide wire can be seen exiting the anterior abdominal wall with the other end emerging from the patient's mouth.

11. Slide the gastrostomy feeding tube, dilator end first, over the end of the guide wire that is exiting the patient's mouth. Apply a water-soluble lubricant to the gastrostomy feeding tube.

12. Firm tension must be applied to both ends of the guide wire

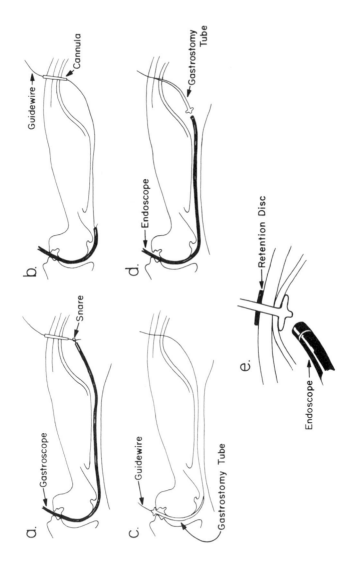

FIG. 1. Percutaneous endoscopic gastrostomy (PEG). See text for details.

as the gastrostomy feeding tube progresses sequentially into the oral pharynx, esophagus, and then the stomach (Fig. 1c).

13. When the tapered tip of the gastrostomy tube begins to exit the anterior abdominal wall, reintroduce the endoscope to observe the gastrostomy catheter exiting the esophagus and monitor the positioning of the internal dome gently against the anterior gastric wall (Fig. 1d).

14. Pull the internal dome firmly but not too tightly. Excess tension should be avoided. If resistance is felt in pulling the gastrostomy catheter through the anterior abdominal wall, enlarge the skin incision. A hemostat may be used to enlarge the opening.

15. Remove the endoscope and cleanse the catheter and wound site.

16. Slide the external retention disc down over the exiting gastrostomy tube (Fig. 1e)

17. Both the internal dome and external disc should allow for rotation.

18. Place an adapter at the end of the gastrostomy tube and attach it to straight drainage.

Procedure 2

With this system, the gastrostomy tube is placed using a modified peel-away sheath over a guide wire. A Foley catheter is then inserted directly through the peel-away sheath. [Prepackaged kits are available from Cook Critical Care, P.O. Box 489, Bloomington, Indiana 47402, (812) 339-2235.] We no longer use this method as we prefer the previously described procedure.

1. After endoscopically selecting and anesthetizing the gastrostomy site, advance a No. 18 gauge needle through the site into the stomach.

2. Insert a flexible J guide wire through the needle into the stomach and remove the needle.

3. Make a small incision adjacent to the guide wire with a No. 11 blade scalpel. This incision should be large enough to allow easy passage of the dilator and sheath.

4. Lubricate the lumen of the modified, 16 French, peel-away

sheath and, with the dilator acting as an obturator, pass the unit over the guide wire (Fig. 2a).

5. Under endoscopic observation, advance as a unit the wire guide, the dilator, and the peel-away sheath into the stomach. Use a rotary motion to facilitate passage.
6. Remove the wire guide and dilator, leaving only the peel-away sheath in the stomach.
7. Lubricate a 14 French Foley catheter and advance it through the sheath until it is seen in the stomach (Fig. 2b).
8. Inflate the Foley balloon with 5 cc water to check the competency of the valve as well as the integrity of the balloon.
9. After confirming that the system is leakproof, peel the sheath away and remove it (Fig. 2c).
10. Bring the Foley catheter into apposition with the anterior abdominal wall by applying slight tension.
11. Suture the catheter to the anterior abdominal wall (Fig. 2d).

Postprocedure

1. Place the gastrostomy tube to straight drainage.
2. Give nothing by mouth except for medications for the next 24 hr. After this period, feeding via the gastrostomy tube may begin, providing that bowel sounds are normal and the patient is afebrile.

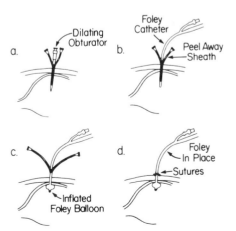

a. Dilating Obturator

b. Foley Catheter — Peel Away Sheath

c. Inflated Foley Balloon

d. Foley In Place — Sutures

FIG. 2. See text for details.

3. Flush the gastrostomy tube with 50 cc of tap water every 4 hr.
4. Change the gastrostomy site dressings daily for 3 days and then remove. This is accomplished by cleansing the wound with hydrogen peroxide and normal saline and then placing slit 4 × 4 gauze pads around the gastrostomy tube. Remove sutures from the external bolster or catheter in approximately 7 days.
5. The patient and family should receive instruction from the nutrition service about further management of the tube feedings at home.

Complications

1. Superficial wound infections.
2. Gastrostomy tube extrusions.
3. Gastrocolic fistula.
4. Pneumoperitoneum.
5. Leakage and peritonitis may occur if the stomach separates from the peritoneum and anterior abdominal wall.
6. Aspiration during the procedure.
7. Fasciitis.
8. Migration of catheter.

BIBLIOGRAPHY

1. Ponsky JL, Gauderer MWL, Stellata TA (1983): Percutaneous endoscopic gastrostomy. *Arch Surg* 118:913–914.
2. Strodel WE, Lemmer J, Eckhauser F, Botham M, Dent T (1983): Early experience with endoscopic percutaneous gastrostomy. *Arch Surg* 118: 449–453.
3. Ponsky JL (1984): Percutaneous endoscopic gastrostomy and jejunostomy: endoscopic highlights. *Gastrointest Endosc* 30:306–307.
4. Russell TR, Brotman M, Norris F (1984): Percutaneous gastrostomy. A new simplified and cost-effective technique. *Am J Surg* 148:132–137.
5. Stassen WN, McCullough AJ, Marshall JB, Eckhauser ML (1984): Percutaneous endoscopic gastrostomy: another cause of "benign" pneumoperitoneum. *Gastrointest Endosc* 30:296–298.
6. Ponsky JL (1985): Endoscopic placement of intestinal tubes. In: *Therapeutic Gastrointestinal Endoscopy*, edited by SE Silvis, pp 94–113. Igaku-Shoin, New York.

7. Ponsky JL (1988): Techniques of percutaneous gastrostomy: a comparison. In: *Techniques of Percutaneous Gastrostomy*, edited by JL Ponsky, p 111. Igaku-Shoin, New York.
8. Strodel WE, Ponsky JL (1988): Complications of percutaneous gastrostomy. In: *Techniques of Percutaneous Gastrostomy*, edited by JL Ponsky, p 63. Igaku-Shoin, New York.
9. Jonas SK, Neimark S, Panwalker AP (1985): Effect of antibiotic prophylaxis in percutaneous endoscopic gastrostomy. *Am J Gastroenterol* 80:438.

33 / Endoscopic Sphincterotomy

Eugene M. Bozymski and Douglas A. Drossman

Endoscopic sphincterotomy is extremely useful in a number of clinical settings. The procedure has virtually replaced surgery for the removal of common duct stones in the patient who has previously undergone cholecystectomy. Endoscopic sphincterotomy is also useful for the removal of common duct stones in the patient with an intact gallbladder who can undergo a laparoscopic cholecystectomy or who is at increased risk for surgery. Another common indication for sphincterotomy is in the preparation for placement of a large stent to relieve neoplastic obstruction of the bile duct.

The solution to the problem of how best to teach and learn endoscopic sphincterotomy has not been adequately addressed. Endoscopic sphincterotomy should not be done by the physician until the skills of selective cannulation of the common bile duct have been mastered. Most often, this level of skill cannot be developed during the usual fellowship period. This training may best be accomplished by having selected fellows stay an additional year in therapeutic endoscopy, or by having gastroenterologists return to the training center for further training in endoscopic sphincterotomy after acquiring more experience with endoscopic retrograde choliangiopancreatography (ERCP).

Indications

1. Gallstones in the common bile duct.
   a. When the gallbladder has previously been removed.
   b. When the gallbladder is present: (i) in the patient at high surgical risk or (ii) in the patient with acute illness (pan-

creatitis, cholangitis) requiring emergency gallstone removal and/or biliary decompression.

   c. In the patient scheduled for or following laparoscopic cholecystectomy.

2. To treat distal common bile duct obstruction: (a) surgical stricture; (b) well-documented ampullary stenosis: (c) ampullary tumor; and (d) choledochocele.
3. Preliminary to the placement of common bile duct stents.
4. Preliminary to choledochoscopy.
5. Treatment of sump syndrome.
6. Treatment of carcinoma of the ampulla of Vater for patients who are not candidates for surgery.

Contraindications

Absolute

1. Impossible access to the papilla (e.g., gastric obstruction).
2. Inadequate training, equipment, or support personnel.

Relative

1. Coagulopathy.
2. Large stone size (>15 mm).
3. Long stricture.
4. Marked portal hypertension.
5. Poor patient cooperation.

Preparation

1. Examine the patient and review the clinical data and laboratory studies to be certain that endoscopic sphincterotomy is the treatment of choice.
2. Obtain coagulation studies. Discontinue aspirin and sodium warfarin (Coumadin) agents for 7 days prior to the procedure.
3. Send a blood clot to the blood bank for typing and cross-match testing if necessary.
4. Make certain that there is no contrast material in the gastrointestinal tract to obscure the area under evaluation.

5. Obtain informed, written consent.
6. Apply the grounding plate on the patient and check that the circuit in the sphincterotome is functioning properly.
7. Place an intravenous (i.v.) line in the right arm with the fork close to the vein for administering atropine, meperidine, midazolam, and glucagon as needed.
8. Place the patient on preprocedure systemic antibiotics (see Isaacs' chapter, "Medications in the Gastrointestinal Procedure Unit") if cholangitis or obstruction of the biliary tree or infection in the pancreas is suspected.
9. Have the patient lie on the left side with the left arm behind the back, to facilitate the roll to the prone position after insertion of the duodenoscope into the duodenum.

Equipment

1. Duodenoscope.
2. Video system or teaching attachment.
3. A variety of cannulas (1.7 mm × 200 cm) with both blunt and tapered tips.
4. Renografin (meglumine diatrizoate) at concentrations of 60% and 30%.
5. Several different papillotomes are available:
   a. Traction type (Demling-Classen):
      Regular—wire ends 3 to 4 mm from tip.
      Precut—wire ends at tip of papillotome.
      Long nose—wire reenters cannula 3 cm from tip.
   b. Push type (Soma).
   c. Billroth II type—reverse-wire placement.
   d. Needle knife.
6. Balloon catheter and Dormia basket for removing stones and mechanical lithotripter.
7. Electrosurgical generating unit.
8. Patient grounding plate.
9. A fluoroscope with good image intensification on a TV monitoring system with capability for taking spot films.
10. X-ray cassettes.
11. Lead aprons and thyroid shields.
12. Gloves, lubricant, syringes, and needles.

Procedure

The physician performing the sphincterotomy should be versed in the anatomy of the biliary tree and have extensive endoscopic experience and skill in the use of electrocautery techniques. A guiding principle behind sphincterotomy is that the length of the incision be based on the reasons for the procedure. For example, the incision length should be long enough (usually 12–13 cm) to allow passage of the largest stone in the common duct as judged by the cholangiogram (with size corrected for magnification) but not so long that it extends beyond the intraduodenal portion of the common duct. When removing small stones, or when placing stents or treating ampullary stenosis, the incision length may be somewhat smaller. The physician should remain familiar with the power output settings on the electrosurgical generating unit. In our unit the power settings are similar to those we use for polypectomy.

1. Proceed with ERCP to obtain a cholangiogram and, if needed, a pancreatogram. Determine the anatomy of the ampulla of Vater and the puncta and the direction required for insertion of the cannula into the common bile duct. This will greatly assist in guiding the sphincterotome into the common duct.

2. Exchange the cannula for a sphincterotome and pass it into the duodenum.

3. When cannulation is difficult, we first recommend exchanging the cannula for a guide wire and then passing the sphincterotome over the guide wire. While working in the "short-stick" position (see Bozymski's chapter, "Endoscopic Retrograde Cholangiopancreatography"), make certain that the ampulla is close up and properly aligned. Recall the direction of the common bile duct, and with the sphincterotome thus directed, insert it for a short distance into the puncta. Inject some dye to make certain that the sphincterotome is in the common bile duct. Continue to insert the sphincterotome well into the common bile duct.

4. Have the assistant open the sphincterotome (making certain that the wire comes out in the 10 to 2 o'clock position relative to the ampulla of Vater). No more than 1.5 cm of wire should be in contact with the intraduodenal segment of the

common bile duct. The wire should not be too taut. Insert the scope 1 to 2 cm to gently lift the ampulla of Vater into the lumen of the duodenum. This allows for close contact of the wire with all parts of the ampulla and permits a more controlled cut to be made in the longitudinal axis of the intraduodenal portion of the common bile duct.

5. Begin the incision with no more than 1.0 cm of the wire within the ampulla. Bow the wire in the properly flexed position with respect to its tension on the ampulla by manipulating the tip of the scope as well as by changing the up-down lever of the sphincterotome. The exposed wire should not be in contact with the tip of the scope, as this will cause electrical current leakage.

6. If the sphincterotome comes out of the common bile duct, reinsert and check fluoroscopically for placement prior to any actual cutting.

7. Apply short bursts (1–3 sec) of coagulation current while lifting the wire until white coagulated tissue is seen near the wire. If there is a great deal of fluid present, more heat will be required. Following this, apply short bursts of blended cut current to lengthen the incision in 1- to 2-mm increments until the planned length of incision is achieved. Some physicians use only the blended cut current to make their sphincterotomy incisions; however, small quantities of coagulation current minimize the chance of bleeding. Too much coagulation current will increase tissue resistance and prevent a controlled incision.

8. Occasionally, when flexing the sphincterotome within the ampulla of Vater, it will back out into the duodenal lumen. Halt this process by having the assistant decrease the flex of the sphincterotome wire and then reinsert the wire. If the incision is being made too rapidly, the assistant should decrease the flexion on the sphincterotome. If bleeding occurs, follow with a little coagulation current along the edges of the cut. Most bleeding is clinically insignificant. With rapid bleeding, the endoscopist may try tamponading with a balloon catheter or injecting 1:10,000 epinephrine into the bleeding area.

9. If on occasion the sphincterotome will not advance into the common bile duct, several maneuvers may be tried:
   a. Make to-and-fro lateral movements of the sphincterotome within the common duct while exerting gentle forward pressure with the right hand.
   b. Make up-and-down movements with the left thumb on the endoscope elevator while advancing the sphincterotome.
   c. Reposition the scope tip to recannulate from a different orientation relative to the papilla.
   d. Wedge the sphincterotome tip at the superior margin of the papillary orifice and fix this position with firm upward pressure of the elevator. Following this, slowly withdraw the endoscope to straighten the angle of the sphincterotome's entry.
   e. On rare occasions, make a small precut to introduce the sphincterotome into the common bile duct (this procedure is associated with a higher complication rate and should not be done until the physician is experienced in sphincterotomy).
   f. At times the sphincterotome can be advanced fluoroscopically by moving the tip of the sphincterotome into a more favorable position within the lumen of the common duct rather than along its wall. Insert the sphincterotome only for very short distances before fluoroscopically checking sphincterotome position to avoid possibly placing the sphincterotome too far into the pancreatic duct.

10. Compare the size of the stones (corrected for magnification) as seen on the cholangiogram with the length of the sphincterotomy using the size of the duodenoscope as a reference measurement. If the sphincterotomy length is considered large enough to permit stone passage, insert a balloon catheter into the common bile duct above the stone; inflate it and pull it down into the duodenal lumen with the stone before it. When the common bile duct is greatly dilated, the stones may slide alongside the balloon into the more proximal common bile duct. When this occurs, try to capture the stones with a biliary basket (Fig. 1). Again, be certain that the

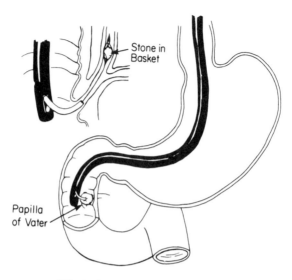

FIG. 1. Gallstone removal with basket.

sphincterotomy size is larger than the entrapped stone. If basket retrieval is to be attempted, we recommend that stone-crushing baskets be available. If the balloon readily passes through the sphincterotomy and is larger than the largest stone, terminate the procedure and await spontaneous passage of the stones. The stool can be strained over the ensuing days to retrieve the stones.

11. If any stones remain at the end of the procedure, place a nasobiliary tube (see Bozymski's chapter, "Endoscopic Biliary Decompression: Nasobiliary Tube") for decompression and reevaluate in several days.

12. Because of the reverse direction of approach, sphincterotomy is particulary difficult (but not impossible) in the patient with a Billroth II gastrectomy and is associated with a higher complication rate. While forward-viewing endoscopes have been recommended to permit better visualization, cannulation is problematic, since there is no elevator. Recently, the use of the wide-angle side-viewing endoscopes and Billroth II reverse-wire papillotomes has considerably increased the suc-

cess rate. Sphincterotomy is also more difficult if the patient has undergone previous surgery in the duodenal area such as a choledochoduodenostomy or if there is anatomic distortion by tumor, and may be more difficult if periampullary diverticula are present.

Postprocedure

1. Monitor vital signs for 1 hr in the recovery area.
2. Clear-liquid diet for the remainder of the day and then resume regular diet.
3. Bathroom privileges for 6 hr post procedure; then ambulation ad lib.
4. Maintain an i.v. with D_5W.
5. Determine hematocrit or serum amylase within 24 hr as clinically indicated.
6. If there has been extensive manipulation of the common bile duct and residual stones are present, broad-spectrum antibiotics are continued.

Complications

The complication rate ranges up to 10%, with a 30-day mortality of up to 1.4%. A 1% to 2% incidence of restenosis is reported. These rates vary directly with the age of the patient and inversely with the experience of the endoscopist. The complication and mortality rates for surgery with common bile duct stone removal are two to three times greater.

Immediate

1. Bleeding (up to 5%). Most severe episodes occur immediately.
2. Perforation (up to 2%), due to improper cut angle, long incision, small common bile duct, or forceful stone pulling.
3. Stone impaction.
4. Oversedation.

Delayed

1. Cholangitis (up to 5%). Requires repeat effort to remove the stones or achieve tube drainage.
2. Pancreatitis (up to 3%).
3. Bleeding.
4. Cholecystitis (if gallbladder present).
5. Impaction of stone in distal duct or distal ileum.

BIBLIOGRAPHY

1. Zimmon DS (1984): Devices and techniques for endoscopic sphincterotomy. Editorial. *Gastrointest Endosc* 30:214–215.
2. Siegel JH (1983): Instrumentation evaluation: endoscopic retrograde cholangiopancreatography and endoscopic sphincterotomy. *Gastrointest Endosc* 29:42–44.
3. Silvis SE, Vennes JA (1985): Endoscopic retrograde sphincterotomy. In: *Therapeutic Gastrointestinal Endoscopy*, edited by SE Silvis, pp 198–240. Igaku-Shoin, New York.
4. Geenen JE (1982): New diagnostic and treatment modalities involving endoscopic retrograde cholangiopancreatography and esophagogastroduodenoscopy. *Scand J Gastroenterol Suppl* 77:93.
5. Safrany L, Cotton PB (1982): Endoscopic management of choledocholithiasis. *Surg Clin North Am* 62:825.
6. Neoptolemos JP, Carr-Locke DL, London NJ, et al (1988): Controlled trial of urgent endoscopic retrograde cholangiopancreatography and endoscopic sphincterotomy versus conservative treatment for acute pancreatitis due to gallstones. *Lancet* 2:979–983.
7. Cotton PB, Vallon AG (1981): British experience with duodenoscopic sphincterotomy for removal of bile duct stones. *Br J Surg* 68:373.
8. Huibregtse K, Kimmey MB (1991): Endoscopic retrograde cholangiopancreatography, endoscopic sphincterotomy and stone removal, endoscopic biliary and pancreatic drainage. In: *Textbook of Gastroenterology*, edited by T Yamada, DH Alpers, C Owyang, DW Powell, FE Silverstein, pp 2266–2292. JB Lippincott Company, Philadelphia.

34 / Endoscopic Biliary Decompression: Nasobiliary Tube

Eugene M. Bozymski

Although there are now many ways to achieve decompression of an obstructed biliary tree, the advantages of using the nasobiliary tube are: (a) it is relatively simple to insert; and (b) once in place, cholangiograms may be obtained at any time to check the status of the biliary system. Additionally, the nasobiliary tube may be used to perfuse monooctanoin in selected cases in which common bile duct stones are refractory to removal.

Indications

Nasobiliary drains are used for temporary decompression of an obstructed or partially obstructed common bile duct. Examples include (a) retained stones present after endoscopic sphincterotomy, and (b) decompression of a biliary stricture (e.g., pancreatic mass) prior to surgery.

Contraindications

There are no absolute contraindications, except for technical inaccessibility of the ampulla of Vater.

Preparation

1. Administer broad-spectrum antibiotics in the periprocedure period. An aminoglycoside and a cephalosporin (or a third-generation cephalosporin with *Pseudomonas* coverage) are appropriate.

242 GASTROENTEROLOGIC PROCEDURES

2. Perform an endoscopic retrograde cholangiopancreatogram (ERCP) (see Bozymski's chapter, "Endoscopic Retrograde Cholangiopancreatography").

Equipment

1. Same equipment as that used for an ERCP (see Bozymski's chapter, "Endoscopic Retrograde Cholangiopancreatography").
2. Select any of several nasobiliary catheters (5–7 French, 250–300 cm length) and guide wires as clinically indicated.
3. Silicone lubricant.
4. A small Foley catheter or nasogastric tube for changing the oral biliary catheter into a nasobiliary catheter.

Procedure

1. Initially, we modify our standard blunt-tipped ERCP cannula by enlarging its opening to approximately a No. 18 gauge needle size. Alternatively, a slightly larger ERCP cannula may be used.
2. Cannulate the common bile duct and using fluoroscopic guidance, slide the catheter into an intrahepatic duct.
3. Insert a guide wire of at least 300 cm in length through the ERCP cannula into an intrahepatic radicle. This is facilitated by initially placing a drop of silicone lubricant over the guide wire or using a "slippery" guide wire.
4. Carefully remove the ERCP catheter while maintaining the guide wire deep within the biliary radicle. Gradually retract the catheter as an assistant simultaneously feeds the guide wire into the channel. Monitor fluoroscopically to maintain position of the guide wire.
5. If the guide wire does not slide readily through the standard (5 French) ERCP cannula, a 6 or 7 French cannula may be used. Alternatively, place a Soehendra dilating biliary catheter into the common bile duct and insert the guide wire through this and then remove the Soehendra dilating catheter.

6. Insert the nasobiliary catheter over the guide wire. It is helpful if the guide wire and catheter are of different colors. Keep the guide wire tight and lubricate it with silicone lubricant.

7. Keep the tip of the endoscope very close to the ampulla of Vater so that forward pressure will be directed upward into the common bile duct rather than downward into the duodenum, thus avoiding forming a loop within the duodenum. Monitor the advancement of the tube via fluoroscopy.

8. Manipulate the elevator repeatedly in the upward direction to maintain the progress of the nasobiliary catheter as it proceeds up the proximal bile duct.

9. Using fluoroscopic guidance, pull back the guide wire into the nasobiliary catheter to a point several centimeters below the pigtail portion and gradually remove the scope while simultaneously advancing the nasobiliary catheter through the channel at the same rate. With one-to-one movement, the position of the nasobiliary catheter within the common bile duct will not change.

10. Do not remove the endoscope and guide wire until the nasobiliary catheter is in place in the proximal portion of the bile duct.

11. Once the endoscope is removed, adjust the nasobiliary catheter to its proper position in the biliary tree and along the duodenal and gastric wall and then remove the guide wire using silicone lubricant as necessary.

12. The nasobiliary tube now exits from the mouth and, for greater patient acceptance, must be transferred to exit from the nose. Pass a small soft Foley catheter or nasogastric tube through the nose, pick its end up in the pharynx, and pull it out through the mouth. Cut off the excess portion of the nasobiliary tube. Thread the nasobiliary tube up through the Foley catheter that exits out of the mouth into the proximal portion of the catheter that exits the nose. Reduce the slack of the nasobiliary cannula by pulling on it as it emerges through the Foley catheter. Fluoroscopically check the position of the distal end of the nasobiliary catheter (Fig. 1).

13. Attach a Luer-lock syringe to the nasobiliary catheter and connect to a Foley bag for straight drainage.

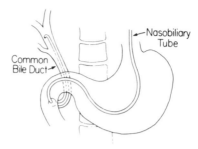

FIG. 1. Position of the nasobiliary drain through the stomach and duodenum into the common bile duct.

Postprocedure

1. Monitor as for ERCP (see Bozymski's chapter, "Endoscopic Retrograde Cholangiopancreatography").
2. Attach the nasobiliary catheter to straight drainage and, using sterile technique, flush once or twice daily.
3. The nasobiliary catheter may be used for repeat cholangiograms as necessary.

Complications

Complications generally relate to the performance of the ERCP (see Bozymski's chapter, "Endoscopic Retrograde Cholangiopancreatography").

BIBLIOGRAPHY

1. Vennes JA (1983): Management of calculi in the common duct. *Semin Liver Dis* 3:162–171.
2. Venu RP, Geenen JE, Toouli J, Hogan WJ, Kozlov N, Stewart ET (1982): Gallstone dissolution using mono-octanoin infusion through an endoscopically placed nasobiliary catheter. *Am J Gastroenterol* 77:227–230.
3. Leuschner U, Wurbs D, Baumgartel H, Helm EB, Classen M (1981): Alternating treatment of common bile duct stones with a modified glyceryl-1-monooctanoate preparation and bile acid-EDTA solution by nasobiliary tube. *Scand J Gastroenterol* 16:497–503.

4. Martin DF, McGregor JC, Lambert ME, Tweedle DEF (1989): Pernasal catheter perfusion without dissolution agents following endoscopic sphincterotomy for common duct stones. *Br J Surg* 76:410–411.
5. Wurbs D, Phillip J, Classen M (1980): Experiences with longstanding nasobiliary tube in biliary disease. *Endoscopy* 12:219–223.
6. Siegel JH (1985): Endoscopic decompression of the biliary tree. In: *Therapeutic Gastrointestinal Endoscopy*, edited by SE Silvis, pp 241–268. Igaku-Shoin, New York.
7. Soehendra N, Reynders-Frederix V (1980): Palliative bile duct drainage: a new endoscopic method of introducing a transpapillary drain. *Endoscopy* 12:8–11.
8. Palmer KR, Hofmann AF (1986): Intraductal monooctanoin for the direct dissolution of bile duct stones: experience in 343 patients. *Gut* 27:196–202.
9. Kozarek RA, Braydo CM, Harlan J, Sanowski RA, Cintora I, Kovac A (1985): Pseudocysts. *Gastrointest Endosc* 31:322–328.

35 / Endoscopic Biliary Decompression: Endoprostheses

Eugene M. Bozymski and Douglas A. Drossman

Endoscopic placement of endoprostheses or stents is a low-risk alternative to operative or percutaneous decompression of obstructing bile duct lesions. This procedure is the preferred treatment for the palliation of obstructing malignant pancreatic or biliary tumors, with a success rate of 70% to 90%.

Endoprostheses are available in a variety of shapes, lengths, and diameters. They range from single- and double-pigtail types to straight stents with side flaps (Amsterdam) (Fig. 1) which offer a greater flow rate. Endoprostheses up to 7 French can be placed through the standard duodenoscope (2.8-mm channel), whereas the larger duodenoscope (4.2-mm channel) is necessary for placement of the 10 and 11.5 French endoprostheses. The smaller prostheses are easier to place but become clogged relatively quickly, and recent data suggest that the rate of cholangitis is higher (34% versus 5%). The larger prostheses are therefore generally preferred, and require a sphincterotomy and the use of a coaxial system with an intermediate-size catheter threaded between the guide wire and stent/pusher system.

Indications

1. To alleviate obstructive jaundice secondary to:
   a. Pancreatic cancer.
   b. Periampullary cancer.
   c. Biliary cancer.
   d. Metastatic cancer.
2. In certain clinical settings, to alleviate obstructive jaundice secondary to benign strictures:

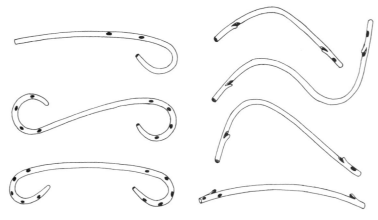

FIG. 1. A variety of endoprostheses.

   a. Chronic pancreatitis.
   b. Postsurgical stricture.
   c. Sclerosing cholangitis.
3. To provide biliary decompression and prevent impaction after sphincterotomy and attempted extraction when gallstones remain in the common bile duct.
4. To provide biliary drainage when a distal common duct fistula exists.

Contraindications

1. See also the chapter by Bozymski and Drossman, "Endoscopic Sphincterotomy."
2. Obstruction due to multiple intrahepatic strictures.

Preparation

1. Generally, the same preparation as is necessary for endoscopic retrograde cholangiopancreatography (ERCP) and sphincterotomy (see chapters by Bozymski, "Endoscopic Retrograde Cholangiopancreatography," and Bozymski and Drossman, "Endoscopic Sphincterotomy").

2. Broad-spectrum antibiotic coverage (e.g., aminoglycoside and a cephalosporin or a third-generation cephalosporin with *Pseudomonas* coverage) is usually indicated (see Isaacs' chapter, "Medications in the Gastrointestinal Procedure Unit").

3. It is essential that the surgical and radiologic consultants be involved in deciding on the course of treatment. We also recommend that the radiologist be in attendance or readily available during the procedure.

Equipment

The equipment is the same as that required for ERCP and endoscopic sphincterotomy (see chapters by Bozymski and by Bozymski and Drossman, as cited above). In addition, the following should also be available:

1. A wide selection of endoprostheses of varying diameters (7, 10, and 11.5 French) and lengths (5–15 cm measured between the flanges) may be used (Fig. 1). These are available with accompanying guide wires (400 cm or greater recommended), guide catheters (350 cm), and pusher cannulas of various colors.

2. Dilating biliary catheters (e.g., Soehendra type) of varying diameters (5–12 French).

3. Snare or grasping forceps to retrieve an endoprosthesis.

Procedure

Successful endoprosthesis placement requires close coordination among the physician and at least two assistants during the procedure: One assists with the equipment and the other monitors the patient.

1. Perform a diagnostic ERCP (See Bozymski's chapter, "Endoscopic Retrograde Cholangiopancreatography").

2. After obtaining the cholangiogram, choose the appropriate-length endoprosthesis, depending on the evident pathology and anatomic configuration of the common bile duct. We use the straight endoprosthesis with side flaps (Amsterdam) most often. The length of the endoprosthesis is determined by the

distance from 2 cm above the stricture to 1 cm below the opening of the bile duct in the duodenum (adjusting for radiographic magnification). The method of inserting an endoprosthesis is similar to that used for inserting a nasobiliary tube (see chapter by Bozymski, "Endoscopic Biliary Decompression: Nasobiliary Tube").

3. Perform a 5-mm sphincterotomy (see chapter by Bozymski and Drossman, "Endoscopic Sphincterotomy") if a large endoprosthesis is to be used or if the anatomic situation requires one prior to the placement of the endoprosthesis.

4. Cannulate the common bile duct. Advance a guide wire (0.035 in. × 400 cm) through the cannula so it is well into the intrahepatic bile radicles.

5. If traversing the narrowed area with a stent may be difficult, thread a Soehendra biliary dilating catheter over the guide wire and across the lesion until the segment is dilated to the size of the endoprosthesis to be used.

6. Based on anatomy and clinical need, choose the appropriate endoprosthesis.

   a. *Small endoprosthesis (7 French).* Mount the tapered end of the endoprosthesis directly onto the guide wire and advance it into the endoscope using a pushing catheter of the same size, but of a different color than the endoprosthesis.

   b. *Larger endoprosthesis (10 and 11.5 French).* The larger endoprostheses require a larger duodenoscope (4.2-mm channel) and are inserted using a coaxial system. Thread a 6.5 French inner catheter over the guide wire and advance it through the stricture. If needed, dilators can be threaded over the catheter. Following this, slide the endoprosthesis (tapered end first) over the taut inner catheter and advance it into the endoscope.

7. Once the endoprosthesis is in the shaft of the endoscope, it cannot be retracted. Therefore, it is important to have the tip of the scope very close to the ampulla of Vater so that when the endoprosthesis comes into view, it is close enough to the puncta to be directed cephalad without pulling the guide wire back into the duodenum.

8. As the prosthesis emerges from the scope (recognized by its different color), continue to advance it into the common bile

duct as the assistant pulls back on the guide wire (or guide wire/inner catheter system). Use the elevator frequently to lift the endoprosthesis as it is advanced. This will keep proper angulation of the prosthesis relative to the common bile duct. Silicone lubricant should be used to decrease friction between the guide wire and the pusher cannula. If the direction of force of the pusher tube exerted on the endoprosthesis is incorrect, the guide wire will form a loop in the duodenum and will begin to back out of the common bile duct. This problem can be minimized by monitoring the procedure fluoroscopically and by having the assistant keep the guide wire taut. If looping occurs, have the assistant gently pull back on the guide wire to reduce the slack. Fluoroscopically monitor the distal end for any slippage that might occur.

9. When the prosthesis is securely in place, have the assistant remove the guide wire (and catheter) as you hold the prosthesis in place by using forward pressure on the pusher. As the guide wire exits the duodenal end of the endoprosthesis, the pusher rod and the endoprosthesis are separated. Final adjustment of the tip of the endoprosthesis can be made by using the pusher cannula that is seen at the tip of the endoscope.

10. Observe the bile flow and fluoroscopically recheck the placement of the stent before removing the endoscope.

11. On certain occasions, it is difficult to obtain guide wire access into the common bile duct beyond (proximal to) the stricture. In this situation, the obstructed bile duct is drained percutaneously by radiologic technique. At a later time, an endoscopically placed prosthesis can be placed with assistance from the interventional radiologist. A guide wire can be passed through the stricture distally via the percutaneous route and then grasped by the endoscopist with a snare or basket passed through the endoscope. After the guide wire is pulled back through the endoscopy channel, the inner guide catheter and stent can be placed in the usual fashion. Alternatively, a basket can be passed percutaneously to grasp the endoscopically placed guide wire.

12. Depending on the clinical situation, we recommend that the

stent be replaced between 4 and 6 months to prevent later complications, such as clogging or fracture.

Postprocedure

1. Monitor the patient's status as per sphincterotomy and nasobiliary stent placement (see chapters by Bozymski and Drossman, "Endoscopic Sphincterotomy," and Bozymski, "Endoscopic Biliary Decompression: Nasobiliary Tube").
2. Obtain serial liver chemistries to monitor the adequacy of the biliary decompression.
3. Continue intravenous antibiotics for 24 hr.
4. The patency of the endoprosthesis may later be determined with radionuclide scanning. Alternatively, another ERCP can be done by inserting a cannula into the tip or alongside the endoprosthesis and injecting contrast material.

Complications

The complication rate ranges from 5% to 30%, with a mortality of up to 1%, depending on the skill of the physician, the size of the endoprosthesis (fewer complications with larger stents), and the location (fewer complications with distal lesions) and number of obstructing lesions. This compares to a surgical mortality up to 20% following surgery for malignant biliary obstruction.

Early Complications

1. Cholangitis (3% distal lesions, 10% proximal lesions).
2. Dislocation.
3. Hemobilia.
4. Perforation.

Late Complications

1. Stent migration (2–5%).
2. Clogging of tube (20–35% within 6 months).
3. Cholangitis.
4. Liver or pancreatic abscess.

5. Fracture of endoprosthesis.
6. Cholecystitis.
7. Perforation.

BIBLIOGRAPHY

1. Laurence BH, Cotton PB (1980): Decompression of malignant biliary obstruction by duodenoscopic intubation of bile ducts. *Br Med J* 280: 522–523.
2. Huibregtse K, Tytgat GN (1982): Palliative treatment of obstructive jaundice by transpapillary introduction of large bore bile duct endoprosthesis. *Gut* 23:371–375.
3. Huibegtse K, Katon RM, Cove PP, Tytgat GNJ (1986): Endoscopic palliative treatment in pancreatic cancer. *Gastrointest Endosc* 32:334–338.
4. Siegel JH (1985): Endoscopic decompression of the biliary tree. In: *Therapeutic Gastrointestinal Endoscopy*, edited by SE Silvis, pp 241–268. Igaku-Shoin, New York.
5. Huibregtse K, Kimmey MB (1991): Endoscopic retrograde cholangio-pancreatography, endoscopic sphincterotomy and stone removal, endoscopic biliary and pancreatic drainage. In: *Textbook of Gastroenterology*, edited by T Yamada, DH Alpers, C Owyang, DW Powell, FE Silverstein, pp 2266–2292. JB Lippincott Company, Philadelphia.
6. Geenen JE, Venu RP (1987): Endoscopic management of biliary obstruction. In: *Techniques in Therapeutic Endoscopy*, edited by J Waye, J Geenen, D Fleischer, pp 6.1–6.19. WB Saunders Company, Philadelphia.
7. Robertson DAF, Hacking LN, Birch S, et al (1987): Experience with a combined percutaneous and endoscopic approach to stent insertion in malignant obstructive jaundice. *Lancet* 2:1449.
8. Kerr RM, Gilliam JH (1988): The team approach to biliary tract intervention: current status of combined percutaneous-endoscopic techniques. *Gastrointest Endosc* 34:432–434.

36 / Colonoscopic Polypectomy

Douglas A. Drossman

Colonoscopic polypectomy is a procedure that is diagnostic; therapeutic; cost-effective, when compared to surgery; and very likely prophylactic for colon cancer (1). [*Note*. All information in Drossman's chapter, "Colonoscopy," applies here. More detailed discussion of polypectomy technique can be found elsewhere (2–5).]

Indication

Removal of colonic polyps greater than 0.5 cm not believed to be invasive polypoid carcinomas. Removal of smaller polyps should be decided on an individual basis.

Contraindications

1. Evidence of a bleeding or coagulation disorder.
2. No available surgical backup for large polyps.
3. Poor bowel preparation.
4. Poor general medical condition of the patient.

Equipment

1. Colonoscope.
2. Coagulator and grounding plate.
3. Colon polyp snare, handle, and sheath; not biopsy forceps.
4. Retrieval instrument (optional).

Preparation

Colonoscopic polypectomy is now routinely performed on an outpatient basis; however, we would recommend overnight hospitalization if the polyp or stalk is large or if complications arise during the procedure.

1. Explain the reasons for the procedure, possible complications, and alternative therapy. Obtain written consent.
2. Test the coagulation equipment to be certain it is in working order.
3. Start an intravenous (i.v.) line and administer meperidine and midazolam as needed.
4. Check the patient's prothrombin time, platelet count, and hematocrit. (For patients with no historical reason for a bleeding disorder, the decision for ordering the tests may be made on an individual basis.)
5. Give subacute bacterial endocarditis (SBE) prophylaxis if indicated (see Isaacs' chapter, "Medications in the Gastrointestinal Procedure Unit").

Procedure

1. Perform a complete colonoscopy (see Drossman's chapter, "Colonoscopy").
2. Attach the ground plate to the patient's thigh.
3. Set the power level based on the manufacturer's recommendations and prior experience with your electrosurgical unit. More power and coagulation time are needed:
   a. For larger polyps.
   b. When there is greater tissue resistance (occurs with dessication during coagulation).
   c. A larger-diameter snare wire is used.
   d. There is less traction on the stalk.
   e. When pure coagulation, rather than blended (cutting and coagulation), current is used.
   For average-sized polyps (1–2 cm), we usually perform polypectomy with a coagulation setting of 2½ to 3 using a 0.42-mm Olympus snare and the Valley Lab Model SSE2 coagulator. If the stalk is very thick or if the snare cannot be

pulled through easily, we may alternate between coagulation and brief bursts of cutting current. Use of pure cut increases the risk of bleeding complications.

4. Identify the polyp and determine if it is pedunculated or sessile. If this cannot easily be determined, manipulate the polyp or reposition the patient to obtain optimal visualization. Be certain there is no excess stool, mucus, or fluid present in the area.

5. If the stalk is large (> 1 cm) or has conical or converging folds, pre-injection of the stalk with 1 ml of a 50% mixture of 1:10,000 epinephrine will reduce the likelihood of a bleeding complication (5).

6. Insert the snare catheter and advance through the colonoscope. Push out the wire to form a loop. Lasso the polyp and place the "V" of the snare on the stalk closer to the head of the polyp than the bowel wall. Ideally, the axis of the stalk should be the same as the snare, in the 6 o'clock position (Fig. 1).

7. Slowly tighten the snare around the stalk, being certain that the head of the polyp or bowel mucosa is not caught and that there is no contact of the polyp head with the opposite wall of the colon. The polyp head should start to turn a dusky blue.

8. Briefly coagulate (¼–½ sec) and observe for a white area of burn on the stalk.

9. Coagulate while pulling the snare through. There should be a smooth but gradually resistive response. If a great deal of resistance is experienced, stop and reexamine for proper positioning of the snare and for blanching of the stalk. Do not pull through without coagulation!

10. If the polyp head unavoidably makes contact with the opposite wall, gently move the catheter back and forth during coagulation to maximize the area of burn contact.

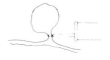

FIG. 1. Snare placement for polypectomy.

11. In 2 or 3 sec, the snare will "snap" when the wire is pulled through the stalk. Observe the stalk for bleeding or excess burn.
12. Remove the polyp by suction, snare, or retrieval instrument (Fig. 2).
13. If bleeding occurs and does not stop spontaneously, two techniques may be used:
    a. Resnare the stalk and tamponade for 5 to 10 min. Do not recoagulate with the snare.
    b. Flush 1:10,000 dilution epinephrine through a catheter impacted into the stalk or inject the base of the stalk. This produces a "bleb" in the submucosa around the vessel and usually stops the bleeding.

On rare occasions, selective intraarterial perfusion of vasopressin, angiographic ablation of the feeding vessel, or surgical intervention is required.

Technique for Small Sessile Polyps (< 1 cm)

Snare-Cautery Technique

The snare-cautery technique can be used to lasso the polyp at its base. Gentle tightening will produce a "pseudostalk" that can then be transected. The small arterial supply and the absence of a true stalk with these polyps make the risk of transmural burn or

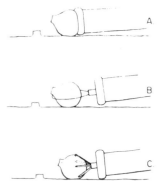

FIG. 2. Method for removal of transected polyps. Polyps may be suctioned (**A**), snared (**B**), or extracted by a pronged retrieval instrument (**C**).

perforation greater than that of bleeding. Therefore, we use a lower coagulation setting (2½). We routinely place a mucus trap in a series with the suction tube to retrieve the polyp.

"Hot-Biopsy" Technique

The hot-biopsy technique can be used for lesions up to 8 mm. There is adequate, but incomplete sampling of tissue. When done effectively, the tissue not in the jaws of the forceps is coagulated. This method is quick and does not cause major bleeding difficulties:

1. Grasp the head of the polyp and pull away from the wall to make a "pseudostalk."
2. Coagulate (2½ setting) and observe for the white burn to extend into but not through the pseudostalk.
3. Do not attempt to burn off the polyp. With the jaws closed, pull off the sample and retrieve it.
4. Observe the area for bleeding or burn.

Technique for Broad-Based Sessile Polyps (1–2 cm)

A sessile polyp less than 2 cm can be removed with one maneuver, providing that the base of the polyp is smaller than its widest diameter.

1. Ensnare and tighten the base of the polyp until it is compressed to no more than 1.5 cm in diameter.
2. Proceed with the polypectomy as previously outlined. A slightly greater current setting may be needed.

Technique for Large Sessile Polyps (> 2 cm)

A clinical decision must be made with regard to the risks and benefits of polypectomy versus those of surgery. The procedure should not be performed if (a) the endoscopist is inexperienced; (b) the polyp appears to contain malignant tissue (ulcerated, friable, irregular contour); (c) the procedure will technically be difficult (poor visualization or ability to manipulate the snare effectively).

1. The polyp is removed in a piecemeal fashion by obliquely encircling one end of the base and placing the "V" of the wire near the top midportion of the polyp (Fig. 3a). No more than 30% of the polyp should be transected with each cut.
2. Coagulate and pull through the tissue.
3. Repeat the procedure at the other end of the polyp (Fig. 3b).
4. A pyramid of tissue will remain. Encircle at least the top half and coagulate it off (Fig. 3c,d).
5. Retrieve all pieces for histopathologic evaluation.
6. If the tissue is benign, colonoscopy should be repeated in 6 to 8 weeks to determine whether further resection is needed. In many cases, the remaining tissue will have sloughed off. If the tissue is malignant, surgery is required.

Postprocedure

1. Fill out a procedure note indicating appearance, size, and location of polyp(s) removed.
2. Send polyp(s) to pathology in individually labeled formalin jars.
3. Check the patient's condition. Note particularly any areas of local abdominal pain or tenderness. Instruct the patient to report back if pain, bleeding, or fever occurs.

Complications (3)

Bleeding (1.7%)

Bleeding complications usually occur when inadequate coagulation is used for pedunculated polyps. It may be observed imme-

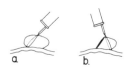

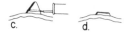

FIG. 3. Removal of large sessile polyp. **a:** Piecemeal removal of polyp. **b:** Procedure repeated at other end of polyp. **c,d:** Top half of polyp is encircled and coagulated off (see text).

diately, within the first 24 hr or in 5 to 7 days (when the fibrin clot falls off). Most bleeding episodes are self-limited and do not require further action.

Perforation (0.3%)

Perforation occurs most often when too much current is applied on sessile polyps or when a portion of adjacent colonic mucosa is transected. Exploratory laparotomy may need to be performed if perforation is clinically detected.

Transmural Burns ("Colon Coagulation Syndrome")

This occurs when the coagulation produces peritoneal inflammation without gross perforation. The patient has localized peritoneal signs, abdominal pain, fever, and leukocytosis within the first 24 hr. Surgery is usually not required. The patient should be given nothing by mouth. Observe for 1 to 2 days and administer i.v. fluids and antibiotics.

Explosion

Since colonic bacteria may produce combustible gases, explosion is a potential hazard. An adequate colonic prep with either cathartics/enemas or lavage solution is sufficient to eliminate this risk (6). We also recommend that carbohydrates be eliminated from the diets of patients about to have a polypectomy.

REFERENCES

1. O'Brian MJ, Winawer SJ, Zauber AG, et al (1990): The National Polyp Study. *Gastroenterology* 98:371–379.
2. Fruhmorgen P (1981): Therapeutic colonoscopy. In: *Colonoscopy: Techniques, Clinical Practice and Colour Atlas*, edited by RH Hunt, JD Waye, pp 199–236. Chapman and Hall, London.
3. Tedesco FJ (1985): Colonoscopic polypectomy. In: *Therapeutic Gastrointestinal Endoscopy*, edited by SE Silvis, pp 269–288. Igaku-Shoin, New York.

4. Waye JD (1987): Gastrointestinal polypectomy. In: *Techniques in Therapeutic Endoscopy*, edited by J Waye, J Geenen, D Fleischer, pp 7.1–7.20. WB Saunders Company, Philadelphia.
5. Williams CB (1990): The 'difficult' polyp. *Can J Gastroenterol* 4:533–536.
6. DiPalma JA, Brady CE, Stewart DL, Karlin DA, et al (1984): Comparison of colon cleansing methods in preparation for colonscopy. *Gastroenterology* 86:856–860.

37 / Unique Aspects of Gastrointestinal Procedures for Pediatric Patients

Martin H. Ulshen

Virtually any gastrointestinal (GI) procedure available for adults can also be performed in infants and children. Withholding a study only because of concern about the patient's size may, in fact, be detrimental to the child's care. On the other hand, some procedures are technically more difficult in children. In addition, even an experienced gastroenterologist may have difficulty if he or she is not comfortable working with children. For these reasons, there may be times when it is best to refer the patient to a physician with expertise in the field of pediatric gastroenterology.

Sedation

Specialty wide standards have not been established for the use of conscious sedation in pediatric gastroenterologic procedures. However, current interest in this topic suggests that a consensus is likely to be developed in the next few years. Procedures should be done under sedation only in an area where the proper equipment is available for resuscitation of the pediatric patient and where individuals familiar with pediatric resuscitation are nearby.

1. The greatest difficulty in working with infants and young children is their inability to comprehend and cooperate.
2. Children old enough to comprehend benefit from an explanation about the procedure in advance and often from a tour of the area where it will be done. Any facility where procedures are done regularly with children should have support from a

play therapist. This therapist can help by reviewing the procedure with the child while he or she acts the part of the physician, using a doll as the patient.

3. Older children often need this kind of introduction to tolerate the less uncomfortable tests, such as small-bowel biopsy and sigmoidoscopy. One may also give an older child the choice as to whether he or she would prefer sedation.

4. The physician must be prepared to spend a greater amount of time performing a procedure in a child than might be necessary in an adult. It is best to explain each step of the procedure immediately before performance and to avoid sudden, unexpected movements.

5. Young children (i.e., < 5 years of age) often need sedation or, very rarely, general anesthesia, depending on the procedure.

6. For the procedures associated with the least discomfort, such as small-bowel biopsy, sigmoidoscopy, or liver biopsy, milder sedation given 45 min or 1 hr before the procedure may be all that is necessary. *The dosage given below is for otherwise healthy children receiving no other medications.*

7. When conscious sedation is used, monitoring of oxygen saturation, pulse, and blood pressure should probably be routine. Under conditions of heavy sedation, a nurse should be available to monitor the patient without preoccupation with the technical aspects of the procedure. In addition, some endoscopists are routinely providing oxygen by nasal cannula during a procedure (2 liters/min).

Oral Medication

If oral medication is desired:

1. Chloral hydrate, 50 mg/kg (maximum 2 g), with diphenhydramine, 1.25 mg/kg (maximum 50 mg); *or*
2. For older children, diazepam, 5 to 10 mg.
3. Oral midazolam has been used effectively in young children.

Intramuscular Medication

If *intramuscular medication* is desired, the following combination works well for small-bowel biopsy: meperidine, 1 mg/kg (maximum 50 mg), and pentobarbital (Nembutal), 5 mg/kg (maximum 100 mg).

For Upper and Lower Gastrointestinal Endoscopy
Children

Intravenous midazolam and meperidine may be administered in a manner similar to the use in adults. Drugs are given slowly while observing the patient's cardiorespiratory status and level of sedation. The effects of meperidine are more easily reversed (with naloxone). Therefore, we tend to use relatively more meperidine. Meperidine is usually given in a dose from 1 to 2 mg/kg. Depending on the length of the procedure, the respiratory status, and the level of consciousness, as much as 3 to 4 mg/kg total dose of meperidine is given occasionally in smaller increments. As in adults, the midazolam dose should be carefully titrated. Generally, the dose of midazolam should be in the range of 0.05 to 0.2 mg/kg, although one should probably not use more than 1 to 2 mg total. A recent consideration is that fentanyl may be a better choice than meperidine (Demerol) because its action peaks more rapidly and is of shorter duration. The starting dose is 1 μg/kg; as with the other intravenous drugs, the dose should be titrated. Intravenous lidocaine has been used when necessary to decrease airway reactivity during upper endoscopy, at a dose of 1 mg/kg.

When sedating a child, one should continuously monitor blood pressure, pulse, and percutaneous measurements of oxygen saturation. A baseline value should be obtained before the procedure for comparison. In addition, measurements should be made after the procedure and at the time of discharge from the unit.

If a child continues to be combative despite heavy sedation, it is safer to do the procedure under general anesthesia with the airway protected. This step is rarely necessary.

Infants

Infants almost never require general anesthesia when upper endoscopy is performed by an individual experienced in examining infants with the newer pediatric endoscopes. Infants under 6 months of age often tolerate upper endoscopy extremely well with light sedation. They object to swallowing the endoscope, but once passed, will often suck on the tube and fall asleep. Up to 2 to 3 years of age, it may be simplest to administer sedation by mouth or intramuscularly. Intravenous administration allows one to titrate the quantity of drug against the requirements of the child.

Procedures in Infants and Children

Upper Gastrointestinal Endoscopy

Endoscopy may be performed with nearly any child from full-term newborn upward, using a pediatric endoscope. Occasionally the instrument will fail to pass through the pylorus in a young infant. Swabbing or spraying the posterior pharynx with local anesthetic can be helpful, but is not absolutely necessary. Biopsies are performed as in adults. Biopsies are especially helpful in evaluating esophagitis because gross appearance of the esopohagus may be misleading, and symptoms are often vague in children. Foreign bodies can be removed from the upper GI tract with the use of grasping forceps or snare. This can be done under general anesthesia or with sedation and the use of an overtube.

Esophageal Dilatation

The indications and contraindications are similar to those in adults. The main limitation is the lack of cooperation that can occur when multiple dilatations are necessary. Ideally, if this is a problem, these dilatations can be done in an ambulatory surgery setting with brief anesthesia. Hurst and Maloney dilators are probably used most often in children. Teenagers generally tolerate this procedure with only local anesthetic. Endoscopic dilatation with Savary-Gilliard bougies can be done under fluoroscopic control in the same manner as performed in adults. Through-the-scope (TTS) balloon dilatation may rarely be necessary initially for very tight strictures.

Sclerotherapy for Esophageal Varices

Sclerotherapy can be performed in the same manner as in adults. Often this procedure can be done in children with intravenous sedation. If the child cannot remain quiet during the procedure, brief anesthesia may be necessary. Sclerotherapy can be performed in infants, although the volume of each injection probably should be reduced to about one-fourth of the adult dose. Early experience suggests that sclerotherapy may be especially beneficial for varices secondary to extrahepatic portal hypertension. The role of sclerotherapy has increased as it has become a temporizing measure while awaiting liver transplantation.

Percutaneous Liver Biopsy

The indications for liver biopsy in infants are somewhat different from those used in adults. The most common reason for liver biopsy in an infant is the evaluation of neonatal cholestasis. The differential diagnosis differs from that of cholestasis in adults. Therefore, the evaluation of these infants should only be done by a physician familiar with this differential and knowledgeable about the studies necessary and treatment. In older children, the most common indication for liver biopsy is chronic hepatitis. Although one cannot expect an infant or child to be cooperative for percutaneous liver biopsy, this procedure can be done safely if adequate sedation is given. As for adults, coagulation studies (including a bleeding time) should be checked before a biopsy is performed. After biopsy, the patient's vital signs should be monitored frequently. Having a patient lie on the right side for 2 hr after the biopsy and then remain at bed rest is standard procedure; however, it is often easiest to keep an infant or young child quiet and calm in his or her mother's arms.

A No. 18 gauge pediatric Menghini needle is available; however, many physicians who perform liver biopsies in infants and children prefer a No. 16 Menghini or Klatskin needle, since the No. 18 needle provides a specimen of less adequate width. The liver biopsy needle is longer than necessary for a child but may be used safely if it is held firmly between the thumb and forefinger 1.5 to 3 cm from the skin when the needle tip is at the liver surface. This provides a guard against excess penetration. The biopsy is performed at the midpoint of upper and lower dullness to percussion or may be performed subcostally if the liver is enlarged at least several centimeters below the costal margin. The procedure is similar to the method in adults, except that it is unrealistic to expect the patient to exhale on command. The biopsy can be timed with the respiratory cycle of the patient while the child is breathing quietly.

Flexible Sigmoidoscopy

In infants, an excellent view of the rectum, and often the sigmoid and descending colon as well, can be obtained with the use of a pediatric upper endoscope inserted as a colonoscope. In children beyond 2 years of age, we tend to use a pediatric or adult colonoscope for flexible sigmoidoscopy.

For young infants, preparation of the colon is usually unnecessary. For older children, one can prepare with medicines from above or below. If the evaluation is for mucosal details (e.g., colitis), we prefer to prepare from above with magnesium citrate or milk of magnesia (2 ml/kg) plus a laxative to stimulate emptying of the rectum, both given the night before the procedure. Alternatively, a balanced electrolyte solution, as described below, can be used; however, it is usually unnecessary to put the child through the unpleasantness of this preparation for an examination limited to the rectosigmoid. The child has a clear-liquid meal the night before and again for breakfast. A tap water or saline solution enema may be adequate alone if the child has loose stools. A Fleet phosphate enema immediately before the procedure works well if the evaluation is for polyps and mucosal detail is not a concern.

Sedation is unnecessary in infants and older children if the examination is limited to the rectum alone; however, pre-schoolers often will not allow any procedure without sedation. For more extensive examination, sedation as described above for minor procedures is appropriate.

Colonoscopy and Polypectomy

Pediatric colonoscopes are available for use in young children, although an adult colonoscope often can be used beyond 2 to 3 years of age. Preparation of the colon is probably best done the night before the procedure with a balanced electrolyte solution given by mouth or nasogastric tube. Younger children will not voluntarily drink an adequate quantity of this solution, and the latter method is usually necessary. Nausea often accompanies the administration of this solution in children, and it is advisable to give metoclopramide (0.1 mg/kg) before the start. The proper volumes of these solutions for size have not been established. As a starting point, we use 1,000 ml/1.73 m^2/hr given over 3 to 4 hr; however, the solution should be continued until the stools are clear. Only clear liquids are allowed for supper and breakfast. As an alternative prep, the child may take only clear liquids by mouth for 48 hr and milk of magnesia on the 2 nights before the procedure. It may be necessary to use tap water or saline enemas on the day of the procedure with this prep. One can be surer that the colon will be adequately cleaned with the balanced electrolyte solution; however, the latter approach avoids the need for hospitalization and nasogastric drip. If the child is having diarrhea, a less stringent prep may be adequate. If the possibility of cautery is anticipated one should avoid natural sweeteners on the morning of the procedure. Sedation is identical to that used for upper endoscopy, although intravenous sedation is often given at a younger age, since this procedure is associated with greater discomfort.

Most colonic polyps in children are juvenile polyps. These polyps tend to autoamputate and do not require routine removal. The indications for polypectomy include significant blood loss, abdominal pain, recurrent intussusception, prolapse, persistent rectal bleeding beyond 6 to 12 months, or removal for diagnostic purposes. However, colonoscopy is used frequently as a primary mode of evaluation of rectal bleeding, and polyps are often identified during this procedure. At that point it seems appropriate to perform a polypectomy even when the above criteria have not been met rather than have the possibility of having to do a colonoscopy later for removal. In addition, parents are often relieved to have the polyp removed despite previous reassurance that it is benign. The method of polypectomy is identical to that used for adult patients.

Colonic Biopsy

Endoscopic biopsy of the colonic mucosa is performed in the same manner as in adults. If a larger or deeper biopsy is required, e.g., for Hirschsprung's disease, suction biopsy can be done safely in any age infant or child, using a Rubin-Quinton tube (4,5). An adequate specimen to diagnose Hirschsprung's disease requires that the depth of submucosa be at least equal to the depth of the mucosa. Therefore, it has been recommended that 15 to 20 mm Hg pressure be applied when doing a suction biopsy for this diagnosis. The biopsy should be done above the distal 1 to 2 cm of rectum but below the peritoneal reflection. Ganglion cells are morphologically immature in infants in the first months of life and can best be identified by an experienced individual.

REFERENCES

1. Ament ME, Christie DL (1977): Upper gastrointestinal fiberoptic endoscopy in pediatric patients. *Gastroenterology* 72:1244–1248.
2. Andrassy RJ, Issacs H, Weitzman JJ (1981): Rectal suction biopsy for the diagnosis of Hirschsprung's disease. *Ann Surg* 193:419–424.
3. Cadranel S, Rodesch P, Peeters JP, Cremer M (1977): Fiberendoscopy of the gastrointestinal tract in children. *Am J Dis Child* 131:41–45.
4. Hargrove CB, Ulshen MH, Shub MD (1984): Upper gastrointestinal endoscopy in infants: diagnostic usefulness and safety. *Pediatrics* 74:828–831.
5. Howard ER, Stamatakis JD, Mowat AP (1984): Management of varices in children by injection sclerotherapy. *J Pediatr Surg* 19:2–5.
6. Shub MD, Ulshen MH, Hargrove CB, Siegal GP, Groben PA, Askin FA (1985): Esophagitis: a frequent consequence of gastro-esophageal reflux in infancy. *J Pediatr* 107:881–884.
7. Vanderhoff JA, Ament ME (1976): Proctosigmoidoscopy and rectal biopsy in infants and children. *J Pediatr* 89:911–915.
8. Yunis EJ, Dibbins AW, Sherman FE (1976): Rectal suction biopsy in the diagnosis of Hirschsprung disease in infants. *Arch Pathol Lab Med* 100:329–333.

9. Casteel HB, Fiedorek SC, Kiel EA (1990): Arterial blood oxygen desaturation in infants and children during upper gastrointestinal endoscopy. *Gastrointest Endosc* 36:489–493.
10. Tolia V, Brennan S, Aravind MK, Kauffman RE (1991): Pharmacokinetic and pharmacodynamic study of midazolam in children during esophagogastroduodenoscopy. *J Pediatr* 119:467–471.
11. Maksoud JG, Goncalves ME, Porta G, Miura I, Velhote MC (1991): The endoscopic and surgical management of portal hypertension in children: analysis of 123 cases. *J Pediatr Surg* 26:178–181.

38 / Small-Bowel Biopsy in Pediatric Patients

Martin H. Ulshen

In general, small-bowel biopsy in a child is similar to biopsy in an adult. Usually, the Carey capsule or pediatric Crosby-Kugler capsule is quicker and easier to use in a child than the Rubin-Quinton tube (1,2). The Carey capsule is simplest, but the pediatric Crosby-Kugler capsule, which is shortest, occasionally passes through the pylorus in a young infant (less than 1 month of age) when the Carey capsule will not.

Indications

1. Diagnosis of any of the diffuse mucosal diseases of small intestine (e.g., gluten-sensitive enteropathy, eosinophilic gastroenteritis, abetalipoproteinemia).
2. Confirmation of disaccharidase deficiency (e.g., congenital sucrase-isomaltase deficiency).
3. Diagnosis of *Giardia* when stool specimens are negative.

Contraindications

1. Bleeding disorder (see Contraindications, item 2 in chapter by Lesesne, "Percutaneous Liver Biopsy").
2. Severe malnutrition with hypoproteinemia and/or hypokalemia.

Preparation

1. Older children should be given nothing by mouth overnight; in young infants, give nothing by mouth for 4 hr only.
2. Sedation may be required in patients up to 6 to 8 years of age

and may be given as needed in older children. Premedications may be given p.o. or i.m. (see the chapter by Ulshen, "Unique Aspects of Gastrointestinal Procedures for Pediatric Patients").

3. Topical anesthesia may be used in patients who are not sedated.
4. Check hematocrit, platelet count, PT, PTT.
5. Explain procedure to family and to child as well, if old enough to understand.

Equipment

1. Carey capsule with cardiac catheter tubing and cardiac catheter straight guide wire (or Crosby-Kugler capsule with similar tubing).
2. Outer bite protection tubing. This is a 10- to 15-cm length of No. 14 French nasogastric tubing that has a longitudinal slit (cut with scissors). This tubing can be placed over the more delicate cardiac catheter tubing for protection during swallowing and can be subsequently removed without disassembly of the capsule and cardiac catheter tubing.
3. Fluoroscope.
4. Suction.
5. Plastic mesh.
6. Forceps.
7. Fine scissors.
8. Aluminum foil.
9. Glass slides.

Procedure

1. Assemble the capsule.
2. Test the capsule.
   a. Carey—be sure the spring is in place and that the capsule moves freely.
   b. Crosby—place rubber glove against ports and trigger with syringe.
3. It is best to swaddle a child who may be uncooperative in addition to providing sedation. Children over 5 to 8 years of age frequently will not require these measures.

4. With the guide wire and outer plastic bite tubing in place, pass the capsule to the posterior pharynx. It is easiest with an uncooperative child to start with the child or infant lying supine. Maintain steady, light pressure on the outer tube and pass this as the child swallows. As an alternative to the use of plastic tubing, one can pass the capsule through a bite block (as used for upper endoscopy). The advantage of this method is that it decreases the risk of the child biting the person performing the test. However, the use of a bite block allows movement of the cardiac catheter tubing in the back of the throat which may cause gagging.

5. Once the capsule is in the esophagus, withdraw the outer bit tube and keep the cardiac catheter tubing against the buccal mucosa with an index finger. Be sure your finger is far enough into the mouth to keep the tube away from the molars. If this is done correctly (and an assistant holds the child's head still), the child cannot bite you or the tubing. Older children or adults may prefer to hold the tubing themselves.

6. Rotate the child to lie on the right side and advance the tubing. Fluoroscope in 1-sec bursts to observe the position of the capsule. It may be necessary to shake an infant up and down gently to have the capsule fall toward the pylorus.

7. Adjust the tubing to position the capsule in the region of the pylorus and apply steady, moderate pressure to the tubing. If the capsule does not pass through the pylorus easily, manipulate the abdomen with a gloved hand to help move the capsule through. A thumb under the capsule pushing cephalad or under the loop of the tubing along the greater curvature may change the relationship of the capsule with the pylorus and allow it to pass through. If there is difficulty, several cubic centimeters of ice water may be passed through to stimulate the antrum to contract and pop the capsule through the pylorus. Metoclopramide premedication can speed up the positioning of the capsule. The dose of metoclopramide is 0.1 mg/kg and can be given orally.

8. Once the capsule has entered the second portion of the duodenum, it may move more quickly if the guide wire is pulled back several centimeters or removed completely.

9. For the Carey capsule: After removal of the guide wire, duodenal contents may be aspirated with light, steady pressure. When this is complete, wash capsule through with about 3 to 5 cc water followed by a similar amount of air. Move the capsule slightly so that mucosa traumatized during aspiration is not at the port. The biopsy is usually taken at the ligament of Treitz. If the Crosby-Kugler capsule is used, a second tubing may be placed over or alongside the cardiac catheter tubing to allow aspiration of fluid. However, fluid cannot be aspirated through the biopsy capsule.

10. To close the Carey capsule, use a 50-ml syringe and apply steady, firm pressure. You can see the capsule close with fluoroscopy. Syringe pressure must be maintained to keep it closed. To close the Crosby-Kugler capsule, pull on the syringe plunger sharply several times.

11. An assistant can remove the tubing and capsule with steady pressure, always being sure the child cannot bite the tubing.

12. When pressure is released, the Carey capsule will pop open, and the biopsy will be on the spring with mucosal side down. The Crosby-Kugler capsule must be opened to retrieve the two biopsy specimens obtained. You can spread the biopsy by gently teasing with the side of a needle (Fig. 1). The specimen will tend to curl up with mucosal side out. Mount mucosa side up on plastic mesh and, if necessary, spread biopsy again. (This is easiest to do if mesh is lying on a glass slide.) With fine scissors, cut off specimen(s) if needed for enzyme

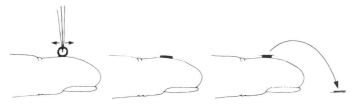

FIG. 1. Orientation of the biopsy specimen prior to fixation. The specimen, which is usually curled as a result of contraction of the cut muscle, must be flattened with the villous side down on the fingertip. This can be done with blunt-tipped pick-up forceps or with the side of a needle. When the specimen is well flattened with the cut side up, a piece of mesh is placed on the cut surface and the specimen is removed from the finger and placed in fixative.

assay. Specimens for disaccharidase assay should be frozen for later analysis. A mucus touch prep for *Giardia* can be obtained by gently touching the biopsy specimen or the Carey capsule spring to a glass slide and immediately placing this slide into fixative for cytologic processing.

Postprocedure

1. Place a brief note in the patient's record that includes the type of procedure, studies for which specimen saved, and amount of fluoroscopy time.
2. When the child is alert, he or she may drink clear liquids and may eat or drink ½ hr later if topical anesthesia has worn off.
3. The patient may leave the hospital within 2 to 3 hr after biopsy.

REFERENCES

1. Carey JB (1964): A simplified gastrointestinal biopsy capsule. *Gastroenterology* 46:550–557.
2. Kilby A (1976): Paediatric small intestinal biopsy capsule with two ports. *Gut* 17:158–159.

39 / Breath Hydrogen Test for Carbohydrate Intolerance

Martin H. Ulshen

The breath hydrogen (H_2) test is a simple, noninvasive study for carbohydrate intolerance that is easily performed. It can be used for infants and children as well as adults. The test is extremely sensitive and, in fact, identifies individuals with asymptomatic carbohydrate malabsorption. For this reason, the results must be interpreted in the context of the clinical setting.

Adult-onset lactose intolerance is an extremely common disorder in adults. About 80% of blacks, Asians, U.S. Indians, Eskimos, and Semites will have lactase deficiency by adult age. This disorder is much less common in northern Europeans and Asian Indians. Those who are symptomatic present with diarrhea, crampy abdominal pain, bloating, flatulence, and occasionally recurrent vomiting. Symptoms may present as early as 5 to 6 years of age; the frequency of this disorder steadily increases through the teens. In contrast to congenital lactase deficiency which is extremely rare, congenital sucrase-isomaltase deficiency is the second most common primary disaccharidase deficiency (well behind adult-onset lactase deficiency). Secondary deficiencies are common after injury to bowel mucosa (especially viral gastroenteritis) and in infants are often symptomatic.

Indications

1. Detection of carbohydrate intolerance, usually a disaccharidase deficiency. This test is most commonly used to identify lactase or sucrase-isomaltase deficiency.
2. Diagnosis of bacterial overgrowth.

Contraindications

None.

Preparation

1. Test for carbohydrate intolerance. Patient should be given nothing by mouth overnight (a minimum of 4–6 hr in infants).
2. Test for bacterial overgrowth. Measure breath H_2 after an overnight fast; the previous night's dinner should be meat and rice bread (avoid other starches).
3. The following conditions may alter the results of a breath hydrogen study: Use of oral antibiotics may be associated with a reduced level, whereas smoking or sleeping during the study may falsely elevate the breath hydrogen level. A small percent of the population lacks the proper colonic flora to produce hydrogen. This situation can be identified by performing a repeat study after ingesting lactulose (a nonabsorbable sugar); if the breath hydrogen is not elevated, the individual is unable to produce hydrogen.

Equipment

1. Breath H_2 analyzer.
2. Breath-sampling device and collection bags.

Procedure

Collection of Breath Samples

Breath samples can be collected with a nasal cannula in an infant or with a mouthpiece and a one-way valve in a child or adult. Collection in infants is timed to manually sample several expirations with the use of a syringe.

Test for Carbohydrate Intolerance

1. A baseline breath sample is collected before administering the carbohydrate.

2. The patient then drinks a 10% to 20% aqueous solution of the carbohydrate under study (1–2 g/kg; maximum of 50 g).
3. Breath samples are collected at intervals of at least 30 min for 1½ to 2 hr; these samples can be analyzed at the time of collection or saved and analyzed simultaneously.

Test for Bacterial Overgrowth

A single fasting sample may be collected. Alternatively, breath hydrogen studies have been done after ingesting glucose (50 g in an adult) or lactulose (10 g in an adult) as a means of identifying bacterial overgrowth.

Postprocedure

Return to previous activities.

Complication

Diarrhea secondary to carbohydrate intolerance.

Interpretation
Carbohydrate Intolerance

Although interpretation of this test is not standardized, most often a rise in H_2 above baseline of greater than 10 to 20 ppm is considered abnormal.

Bacterial Overgrowth

A fasting breath H_2 of greater than 11 ppm is considered abnormal.

BIBLIOGRAPHY

1. Ostrander CR, Cohen RS, Hopper AO, et al. (1983): Breath hydrogen analysis: a review of the methodologies and clinical applications. *J Pediatr Gastroenterol Nutr* 2:525–533.

2. Perman JA, Barr RG, Watkins JB (1978): Sucrose malabsorption in children: noninvasive diagnosis by interval breath hydrogen determination. *J Pediatr* 93:17–22.
3. Perman JA, Modler S, Barr RG, et al. (1984): Fasting breath hydrogen concentration: normal values and clinical application. *Gastroenterology* 87:1358–1363.
4. Levitt MD, Bond JH (1981): Quantitative measurement of lactose absorption and colonic salvage of nonabsorbed lactose: direct and indirect methods. In: *Lactose Digestion: Clinical and Nutritional Implications*, edited by DM Paige, TM Bayless, pp 80–87. The Johns Hopkins University Press, Baltimore.
5. Solomons NW (1981): Diagnosis and screening techniques for lactose maldigestion: advantages of the hydrogen breath test. In: *Lactose Digestion: Clinical and Nutritional Implications*, edited by DM Paige, TM Bayless, pp 91–109. The Johns Hopkins University Press, Baltimore.
6. Barr RG (1981): Limitations of the hydrogen breath test and other techniques for predicting incomplete lactose absorption. In: *Lactose Digestion: Clinical and Nutritional Implications*, edited by DM Paige, TM Bayless, pp 110–114. The Johns Hopkins University Press, Baltimore.
7. Rhodes JM, Middleton P, Jewell DP (1979): The lactulose hydrogen breath test as a diagnostic test for small-bowel bacterial overgrowth. *Scand J Gastroenterol* 14:333–336.
8. Kerlin P, Wong L (1988): Breath hydrogen testing in bacterial overgrowth of the small intestine. *Gastroenterology* 95:982–988.

40 / Esophageal pH Monitoring for Gastroesophageal Reflux

Martin H. Ulshen

Esophageal pH can be monitored to evaluate the presence of gastroesophageal reflux (GER). There are two major methods of monitoring: a continuous, extended study (see also the chapter by Bozymski and Orlando, "Ambulatory Intraesophageal pH Monitoring") or a brief study (Tuttle test). The former method appears to be more reliable. Monitoring requires adequate cooperation to maintain a pH probe in the esophagus for the duration of the study; however, the newer ambulatory monitoring systems allow the patient to continue normal activities during study. Perhaps the greatest weakness in this test is the wide variability in the methods of analyzing the results.

Indications

1. Confirmation of questionable esophageal symptoms or sequelae of GER.
2. Evaluation for the presence of GER in patients with chronic lung disease or recurrent apnea.

Contraindications

None.

Preparation

Patient should be given nothing by mouth for at least 4 hr prior to passing the pH probe.

Equipment

1. Flexible pH microelectrode.
2. Device for measuring and recording pH:
   a. pH meter with recording terminals, patient isolator, strip chart recorder; or
   b. Ambulatory pH meter with microprocessor recording device, microcomputer (or dedicated microprocessor), and printer.

Procedure

1. If necessary, the pH meter is calibrated against buffer (pH 4.0 and 7.0) before inserting the probe.
2. Following application of a local anesthetic solution to the nasal mucosa (4% cocaine works well), the pH probe is passed nasally under fluoroscopic control. The probe is passed into the stomach to document an acid pH and then pulled back to the distal esophagus in the region of the mid-left atrium. The probe should always be at least 2.5 cm above the gastroesophageal junction. The probe lead is immobilized by taping it to the nose at the external naris.
3. *Tuttle test*. A volume of 0.1 N HCl adjusted for size (300 ml/ 1.73 m^2) is given to the patient through a nasogastric tube. Alternatively, apple juice can be given orally in a volume appropriate for size. Esophageal pH is monitored for 10 min with the patient prone or lying on a side. If no GER is seen, abdominal pressure is increased by manual compression, Valsalva, crying, and straight-leg raising for 5 to 10 min.
4. *Extended study*. Recording is done over a period of 12 to 24 hr. The patient maintains a chronologic log of activities, including position (upright, supine, prone), sleep times, mealtimes, and other events (regurgitation, coughing, heartburn, etc.).
5. If a pH meter is used, the meter reading should be rechecked against pH 4.0 buffer at the end of the study.
6. If an ambulatory system is used, the data are fed from the ambulatory microprocessor unit into the computer or dedicated microprocessor.

Postprocedure

Normal diet and activities.

Complications

Virtually none; very low risk of aspiration, as with a small-caliber feeding tube.

Interpretation

Has not been well standardized.

Tuttle Test

Two or more episodes of pH < 4.0 for > 15 sec apiece is a positive result.

Evaluation of Extended pH Study

There are at least three methods for evaluating the extended pH study.

1. Reflux is defined as an episode with pH < 4.0 that lasts at least 15 sec. A weighted score is given for the number of episodes per 12 hr; number of episodes greater than 5 min in duration per 12 hr; longest episode; and total percent of time with esophageal pH < 4.0 during periods awake, asleep, upright, and supine. A final score is derived and compared to an upper limit of normal.
2. Pathologic GER is defined as pH < 4.0 for greater than 10% of the postprandial period.
3. Pathologic GER is defined as pH < 4.0 for greater than 4 min, or a mean of more than 1.5 episodes with pH < 4.0, per hour.

BIBLIOGRAPHY

1. Euler AR, Ament ME (1977): Detection of gastroesophageal reflux in the

pediatric-age patient by esophageal intraluminal pH probe measurement (Tuttle test). *Pediatrics* 60:65–68.

2. Jolley SG, Johnson DG, Herbst JJ, et al (1978): An assessment of gastroesophageal reflux in children by extended pH monitoring of the distal esophagus. *Surgery* 84:16–24.

3. Sondheimer JM (1980): Continuous monitoring of distal esophageal pH: a diagnostic test for gastroesophageal reflux in infants. *J Pediatr* 96:804–807.

4. Winter HS, Madara JL, Stafford RJ, et al (1982): Intraepithelial eosinophils: a new diagnostic criterion for reflux esophagitis. *Gastroenterology* 83:818–823.

Subject Index